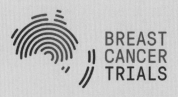

BREAST
CANCER
TRIALS

The Australian Women's Health Diary
funds breast cancer clinical trials research
to save and improve the lives of every
person affected by breast cancer.

Today, tomorrow and forever.

TRIALS SAVE LIVES

A diary of hope

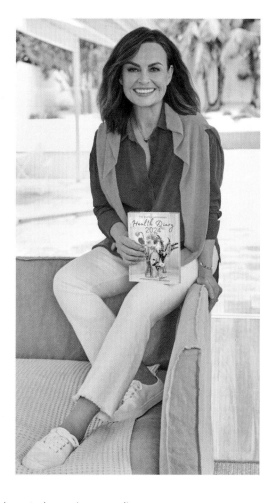

That's why this diary is so important to me. Because of the change it makes and the hope it gives to individuals and families who are impacted by breast cancer.

It's estimated this year that more than 20,000 women and 200 men will receive a diagnosis of breast cancer. That's on top of the 20,000 who were diagnosed last year and the year before and so on, many of whom are still undergoing treatment and facing an uncertain future.

The sheer numbers mean it is rare not to know someone who has had breast cancer, and sadly, who has lost their life. I'm sorry if you have personally been affected.

The funds raised by this diary support the critical work of the researchers at Breast Cancer Trials. Through their clinical trials research, they've already achieved significant breakthroughs, which are today saving many lives.

But they won't stop until every life is saved, until the burdens of fear and uncertainty that accompany every diagnosis are eased, and until every person is protected from breast cancer and its impact.

Through your purchase, you're supporting the research needed to achieve this. You're providing hope for a future where breast cancer no longer has power over lives. Thank you.

And as you use your diary, you'll be reminded of this by the special women whose images appear at the start of each month.

Best wishes for a wonderful year ahead.

LISA WILKINSON

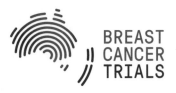

BREAST CANCER TRIALS

Who we are

Breast Cancer Trials is a research charity that conducts national and international clinical trials in breast cancer. Our researchers, located in hospitals throughout Australia and New Zealand, treat and support patients with breast cancer every day. We work with other researchers globally to pool resources, share knowledge and accelerate progress for the benefit of patients and those at risk.

Why we do clinical trials

Because breast cancer isn't the same in every person, it's vital we find tailored treatments and adopt a whole person approach – to save lives, and to improve and protect quality of life, as well as emotional wellbeing.

Our clinical trials, for patients with early-stage or metastatic breast cancer and for those at high risk due to a genetic mutation, can provide patients with access to new breast cancer treatments and strategies not yet widely available. People participate because they may benefit, and because people in the future can benefit from what is learned. The treatments available today are only possible because of this research.

Our research focus

Our priority research areas include stopping breast cancer from occurring in the first place; curing more people with targeted treatment at the time of their first diagnosis to prevent any chance of recurrence of their disease; helping patients with metastatic breast cancer to live longer with good quality of life; and protecting quality of life by reducing the side effects of treatment.

Your support

Our research is made possible thanks to the women and men who participate in our clinical trials and our generous supporters, like you, who donate and buy this diary. Thank you for helping to create a future where breast cancer no longer impacts lives.

SCAN THIS QR CODE TO LEARN MORE.

Calendar
2024

JANUARY

S	M	T	W	T	F	S
	1	2	3	4	5	6
7	8	9	10	11	12	13
14	15	16	17	18	19	20
21	22	23	24	25	26	27
28	29	30	31			

FEBRUARY

S	M	T	W	T	F	S
				1	2	3
4	5	6	7	8	9	10
11	12	13	14	15	16	17
18	19	20	21	22	23	24
25	26	27	28	29		

MARCH

S	M	T	W	T	F	S
31					1	2
3	4	5	6	7	8	9
10	11	12	13	14	15	16
17	18	19	20	21	22	23
24	25	26	27	28	29	30

APRIL

S	M	T	W	T	F	S
	1	2	3	4	5	6
7	8	9	10	11	12	13
14	15	16	17	18	19	20
21	22	23	24	25	26	27
28	29	30				

MAY

S	M	T	W	T	F	S
			1	2	3	4
5	6	7	8	9	10	11
12	13	14	15	16	17	18
19	20	21	22	23	24	25
26	27	28	29	30	31	

JUNE

S	M	T	W	T	F	S
30						1
2	3	4	5	6	7	8
9	10	11	12	13	14	15
16	17	18	19	20	21	22
23	24	25	26	27	28	29

JULY

S	M	T	W	T	F	S
	1	2	3	4	5	6
7	8	9	10	11	12	13
14	15	16	17	18	19	20
21	22	23	24	25	26	27
28	29	30	31			

AUGUST

S	M	T	W	T	F	S
				1	2	3
4	5	6	7	8	9	10
11	12	13	14	15	16	17
18	19	20	21	22	23	24
25	26	27	28	29	30	31

SEPTEMBER

S	M	T	W	T	F	S
1	2	3	4	5	6	7
8	9	10	11	12	13	14
15	16	17	18	19	20	21
22	23	24	25	26	27	28
29	30					

OCTOBER

S	M	T	W	T	F	S
		1	2	3	4	5
6	7	8	9	10	11	12
13	14	15	16	17	18	19
20	21	22	23	24	25	26
27	28	29	30	31		

NOVEMBER

S	M	T	W	T	F	S
					1	2
3	4	5	6	7	8	9
10	11	12	13	14	15	16
17	18	19	20	21	22	23
24	25	26	27	28	29	30

DECEMBER

S	M	T	W	T	F	S
1	2	3	4	5	6	7
8	9	10	11	12	13	14
15	16	17	18	19	20	21
22	23	24	25	26	27	28
29	30	31				

2023

JANUARY
S	M	T	W	T	F	S
1	2	3	4	5	6	7
8	9	10	11	12	13	14
15	16	17	18	19	20	21
22	23	24	25	26	27	28
29	30	31				

FEBRUARY
S	M	T	W	T	F	S
			1	2	3	4
5	6	7	8	9	10	11
12	13	14	15	16	17	18
19	20	21	22	23	24	25
26	27	28				

MARCH
S	M	T	W	T	F	S
			1	2	3	4
5	6	7	8	9	10	11
12	13	14	15	16	17	18
19	20	21	22	23	24	25
26	27	28	29	30	31	

APRIL
S	M	T	W	T	F	S
30						1
2	3	4	5	6	7	8
9	10	11	12	13	14	15
16	17	18	19	20	21	22
23	24	25	26	27	28	29

MAY
S	M	T	W	T	F	S
	1	2	3	4	5	6
7	8	9	10	11	12	13
14	15	16	17	18	19	20
21	22	23	24	25	26	27
28	29	30	31			

JUNE
S	M	T	W	T	F	S
				1	2	3
4	5	6	7	8	9	10
11	12	13	14	15	16	17
18	19	20	21	22	23	24
25	26	27	28	29	30	

JULY
S	M	T	W	T	F	S
30	31					1
2	3	4	5	6	7	8
9	10	11	12	13	14	15
16	17	18	19	20	21	22
23	24	25	26	27	28	29

AUGUST
S	M	T	W	T	F	S
		1	2	3	4	5
6	7	8	9	10	11	12
13	14	15	16	17	18	19
20	21	22	23	24	25	26
27	28	29	30	31		

SEPTEMBER
S	M	T	W	T	F	S
					1	2
3	4	5	6	7	8	9
10	11	12	13	14	15	16
17	18	19	20	21	22	23
24	25	26	27	28	29	30

OCTOBER
S	M	T	W	T	F	S
1	2	3	4	5	6	7
8	9	10	11	12	13	14
15	16	17	18	19	20	21
22	23	24	25	26	27	28
29	30	31				

NOVEMBER
S	M	T	W	T	F	S
			1	2	3	4
5	6	7	8	9	10	11
12	13	14	15	16	17	18
19	20	21	22	23	24	25
26	27	28	29	30		

DECEMBER
S	M	T	W	T	F	S
31					1	2
3	4	5	6	7	8	9
10	11	12	13	14	15	16
17	18	19	20	21	22	23
24	25	26	27	28	29	30

2025

JANUARY
S	M	T	W	T	F	S
			1	2	3	4
5	6	7	8	9	10	11
12	13	14	15	16	17	18
19	20	21	22	23	24	25
26	27	28	29	30	31	

FEBRUARY
S	M	T	W	T	F	S
						1
2	3	4	5	6	7	8
9	10	11	12	13	14	15
16	17	18	19	20	21	22
23	24	25	26	27	28	

MARCH
S	M	T	W	T	F	S
30	31					1
2	3	4	5	6	7	8
9	10	11	12	13	14	15
16	17	18	19	20	21	22
23	24	25	26	27	28	29

APRIL
S	M	T	W	T	F	S
		1	2	3	4	5
6	7	8	9	10	11	12
13	14	15	16	17	18	19
20	21	22	23	24	25	26
27	28	29	30			

MAY
S	M	T	W	T	F	S
				1	2	3
4	5	6	7	8	9	10
11	12	13	14	15	16	17
18	19	20	21	22	23	24
25	26	27	28	29	30	31

JUNE
S	M	T	W	T	F	S
1	2	3	4	5	6	7
8	9	10	11	12	13	14
15	16	17	18	19	20	21
22	23	24	25	26	27	28
29	30					

JULY
S	M	T	W	T	F	S
		1	2	3	4	5
6	7	8	9	10	11	12
13	14	15	16	17	18	19
20	21	22	23	24	25	26
27	28	29	30	31		

AUGUST
S	M	T	W	T	F	S
31					1	2
3	4	5	6	7	8	9
10	11	12	13	14	15	16
17	18	19	20	21	22	23
24	25	26	27	28	29	30

SEPTEMBER
S	M	T	W	T	F	S
	1	2	3	4	5	6
7	8	9	10	11	12	13
14	15	16	17	18	19	20
21	22	23	24	25	26	27
28	29	30				

OCTOBER
S	M	T	W	T	F	S
			1	2	3	4
5	6	7	8	9	10	11
12	13	14	15	16	17	18
19	20	21	22	23	24	25
26	27	28	29	30	31	

NOVEMBER
S	M	T	W	T	F	S
30						1
2	3	4	5	6	7	8
9	10	11	12	13	14	15
16	17	18	19	20	21	22
23	24	25	26	27	28	29

DECEMBER
S	M	T	W	T	F	S
	1	2	3	4	5	6
7	8	9	10	11	12	13
14	15	16	17	18	19	20
21	22	23	24	25	26	27
28	29	30	31			

Personal information

IF FOUND PLEASE CONTACT:

NAME

ADDRESS

STATE   POSTCODE

PHONE NUMBER   MOBILE

EMAIL

IN CASE OF EMERGENCY:

NAME

TELEPHONE   MOBILE

USEFUL TELEPHONE NUMBERS:

DOCTOR   GAS

DENTIST   ELECTRICITY

MECHANIC   WATER

VET   PLUMBER

CHILD CARE   SCHOOL

OTHER IMPORTANT INFORMATION:

Key contacts

NAME

ADDRESS

STATE   POSTCODE

TELEPHONE (H)   (W)

MOBILE   EMAIL

NAME

ADDRESS

STATE   POSTCODE

TELEPHONE (H)   (W)

MOBILE   EMAIL

NAME

ADDRESS

STATE   POSTCODE

TELEPHONE (H)   (W)

MOBILE   EMAIL

NAME

ADDRESS

STATE   POSTCODE

TELEPHONE (H)   (W)

MOBILE   EMAIL

NAME

ADDRESS

STATE   POSTCODE

TELEPHONE (H)   (W)

MOBILE   EMAIL

NAME

ADDRESS

STATE   POSTCODE

TELEPHONE (H)   (W)

MOBILE   EMAIL

Key contacts

NAME

ADDRESS

	STATE	POSTCODE

TELEPHONE (H)   (W)

MOBILE   EMAIL

NAME

ADDRESS

	STATE	POSTCODE

TELEPHONE (H)   (W)

MOBILE   EMAIL

NAME

ADDRESS

	STATE	POSTCODE

TELEPHONE (H)   (W)

MOBILE   EMAIL

NAME

ADDRESS

	STATE	POSTCODE

TELEPHONE (H)   (W)

MOBILE   EMAIL

NAME

ADDRESS

	STATE	POSTCODE

TELEPHONE (H)   (W)

MOBILE   EMAIL

NAME

ADDRESS

	STATE	POSTCODE

TELEPHONE (H)   (W)

MOBILE   EMAIL

Special events 2024

JANUARY

FEBRUARY

MARCH

APRIL

MAY

JUNE

JULY

AUGUST

SEPTEMBER

OCTOBER

NOVEMBER

DECEMBER

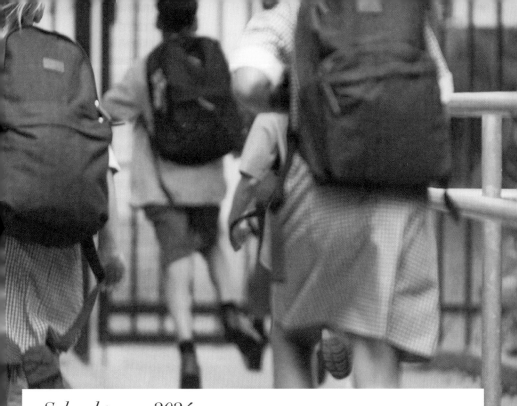

School terms 2024

NEW SOUTH WALES
TERM 1	January 30 – April 12
TERM 2	April 29 – July 5
TERM 3	July 22 – September 27
TERM 4	October 14 – December 20

AUSTRALIAN CAPITAL TERRITORY
TERM 1	January 29 – April 12
TERM 2	April 29 – July 5
TERM 3	July 22 – September 27
TERM 4	October 14 – December 17

QUEENSLAND
TERM 1	January 22 – March 28
TERM 2	April 15 – June 21
TERM 3	July 8 – September 13
TERM 4	September 30 – December 13

VICTORIA
TERM 1	January 29 – March 28
TERM 2	April 15 – June 28
TERM 3	July 15 – September 20
TERM 4	October 7 – December 20

WESTERN AUSTRALIA
TERM 1	January 31 – March 28
TERM 2	April 15 – June 28
TERM 3	July 15 – September 20
TERM 4	October 7 – December 12

NORTHERN TERRITORY
TERM 1	January 29 – April 5
TERM 2	April 15 – June 21
TERM 3	July 15 – September 20
TERM 4	October 7 – December 13

SOUTH AUSTRALIA
TERM 1	January 29 – April 12
TERM 2	April 29 – July 5
TERM 3	July 22 – September 27
TERM 4	October 14 – December 13

TASMANIA
TERM 1	February 7 – April 11
TERM 2	April 29 – July 5
TERM 3	July 23 – September 27
TERM 4	October 14 – December 19

CHECK WITH YOUR SCHOOL FOR DATES OF PUPIL-FREE DAYS

Budget planner 2024

For advice on how best to use this planner, see the Finance chapter in June.

$$$	WEEKLY	MONTHLY	ANNUALLY
INCOME			
Net salary/wage			
Bonuses (after tax)			
Dividends/income from investments			
Interest			
Other			
TOTAL INCOME			
EXPENDITURE			
HOUSEHOLD			
Rent/mortgage			
Council rates			
Water rates			
Power & heating			
Telephone/internet			
House & contents insurance			
Maintenance/repairs			
Other			
PERSONAL			
Groceries			
Clothing			
Child care			
School fees			
Toiletries/cosmetics/haircare			
Mobile phone			
Superannuation			
Other			
LOANS			
Personal loans			
Credit/store cards			
Other			

$$$	WEEKLY	MONTHLY	ANNUALLY
TRANSPORT			
Train/bus/ferry fares			
Car registration			
Car insurance			
Petrol			
Tolls			
Parking			
Other			
HEALTH			
Doctor/dentist/ other specialists			
Health insurance			
Chemist			
Life insurance/ income protection			
Other			
ENTERTAINMENT			
Eating out			
Concerts/movies/ theatre			
Memberships			
Holidays/hobbies			
Newspapers/books			
Streaming services			
Other			
OTHER			
Gifts			
Donations to charity			
Regular investments			
Savings/rainy day fund			
TOTAL EXPENDITURE			
TOTAL INCOME			
INCOME MINUS EXPENDITURE			

DATE OF MY NEXT BUDGET REVIEW   /   /

Health checklist

	LOOKING FOR	HOW OFTEN
Eye examination	Vision loss, general eye health and conditions like glaucoma and cataracts.	From age 65 if you notice vision deterioration. People with family history of glaucoma should have regular, comprehensive eye examinations.
Dental	Gum disease, cavities and general decline in dental health.	Once a year for a check-up, or more often if you have gum issues or plaque build-up.
Hearing	Hearing loss.	When you notice hearing damage or have concerns, or annually for those aged 65 and over.
Bone density scan	Osteoporosis or low bone density.	Consult your GP, especially if you have a family history of osteoporosis or are aged over 50.
Immunisation	Immunity to influenza, Covid-19, tetanus, rubella and others.	As advised by your GP. Flu shots are available yearly, and are free for those aged over 65.
Cervical Screening Test	Signs of the human papillomavirus (HPV) and cervical cancer.	From age 25-74 if you are or have ever been sexually active. If results are normal, continue to be tested every five years thereafter.
STI test	Common sexually transmitted diseases, such as chlamydia, gonorrhoea, syphilis, genital herpes, hepatitis B and HIV.	Every six to 12 months if you're sexually active, have a new partner, frequently change partners, travel to areas with a high prevalence of STIs or have been exposed in the last 12 months.
Breast self-examination	Breast changes, lumps, dimpling or thickening of the skin, nipple change or discharge, pain.	Know the normal look and feel of your breasts. If you notice any new or unusual changes, see your GP, particularly if they persist.
Screening mammogram	Breast lumps or changes not evident to the touch.	Every two years from age 50-74, or annually and earlier if at high risk of breast cancer.
Diabetes screening	Elevated blood glucose levels.	Screening is dependent on your individual risk level. Ask your GP for advice.
Skin check	Spots, moles and freckles which are dry, scaly or have smudgy borders.	Self-check on a regular basis and see your GP about any new or changed skin lesions. Get checked opportunistically if you work outdoors.
Bowel cancer screening	Polyps, other signs of bowel cancer.	Faecal occult blood test every two years from age 50-74, plus a five-yearly colonoscopy. Early testing is available for those deemed to be at moderate risk of bowel cancer; ask your GP.
Blood pressure	High blood pressure, which can increase risk of heart disease and stroke; low blood pressure.	Every two years for adults aged 18 and over, or more often if there's a family history of high blood pressure, stroke, kidney or heart disease.
Cholesterol	High LDL (bad cholesterol) and triglycerides, and low HDL (good cholesterol).	Every five years from age 45, or more often if you're at risk of cardiovascular disease. The results, along with your BP results, will be interpreted by your GP in the context of your overall absolute cardiovascular risk.
Body Mass Index	Healthy weight range and waist measurement.	Every two years by your GP or more if part of an identified or increased risk group.

LAST CHECKED	CONTACT	DATE OF APPOINTMENT	COMPLETED
	For more information, visit cancerscreening.gov.au or call 131 556		
	BreastScreen Australia: 132 050		
	For more information, visit cancerscreening.gov.au or call 1800 118 868		

Aboriginal and Torres Strait Islander people may have different health needs and should discuss these with their GP.

Don't forget

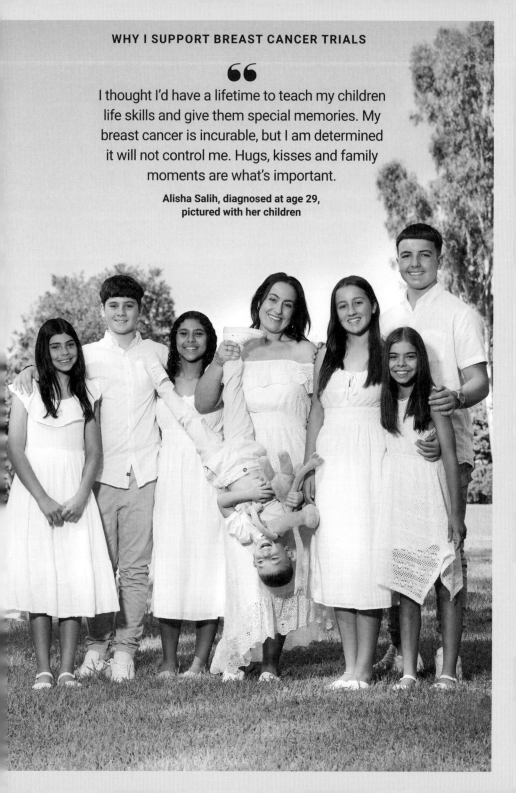

WHY I SUPPORT BREAST CANCER TRIALS

> I thought I'd have a lifetime to teach my children life skills and give them special memories. My breast cancer is incurable, but I am determined it will not control me. Hugs, kisses and family moments are what's important.

Alisha Salih, diagnosed at age 29, pictured with her children

let's talk about
HEALTHY HABITS

It's never too early or too late to make healthy changes, so why not use the beginning of a new year to adopt some positive habits. Try these 10 simple changes for better health and wellbeing.

1 COOK SOMETHING NEW EACH WEEK Diversity is the key to nurturing your body with a variety of beneficial vitamins and nutrients. Set yourself a challenge of cooking one new dinner showcasing a different fresh ingredient each week.

2 LOCK IN IMPORTANT CHECK-UPS Use the Health Checklist at the beginning of this diary and book in all of your medical appointments for the year. Do it in January before life gets busy and you forget.

3 DO AWAY WITH MULTITASKING Trying to do too many things at once can cause feelings of stress and anxiety, and actually makes us less efficient as our focus is fragmented. Instead, allow time in your day for each activity – family, work, exercise, housework, self-care – giving each one your full attention.

4 DO A FINANCIAL AUDIT If you have a home loan, ask your current lender for an annual rate review. Similarly, review your insurance policies and don't be afraid to swap providers to get a better deal.

5 CHECK YOUR POSTURE Sitting slumped on the sofa or hunched at a desk can cause muscle and joint pain,

headaches, digestive issues and poor circulation. Take a moment to straighten your back, tuck in your stomach, uncross your legs and place your feet flat on the floor.

6 FLOSS EVERY DAY You may be in the habit of brushing your teeth twice a day, but do you also floss? Flossing is an essential part of dental hygiene and helps remove food and bacteria trapped between teeth. Ask your dentist for a demonstration if you're unsure of the best technique, or look for easy-to-use dental floss picks.

7 RECYCLE FOOD WASTE Compost bins and worm farms offer an eco-friendly way to dispose of food scraps and make free fertiliser for your garden and plants. Apartment dwellers can join in with small benchtop caddies or by setting up a communal worm farm within their complex.

8 EXERCISE YOUR PELVIC FLOOR Doing regular Kegel exercises will strengthen your pelvic floor muscles and can help prevent incontinence. Squeeze and lift the muscles around your anus and vagina as if you're trying to stop passing wind, then release. You can do these exercises in the car, standing in a queue or while waiting to cross the road.

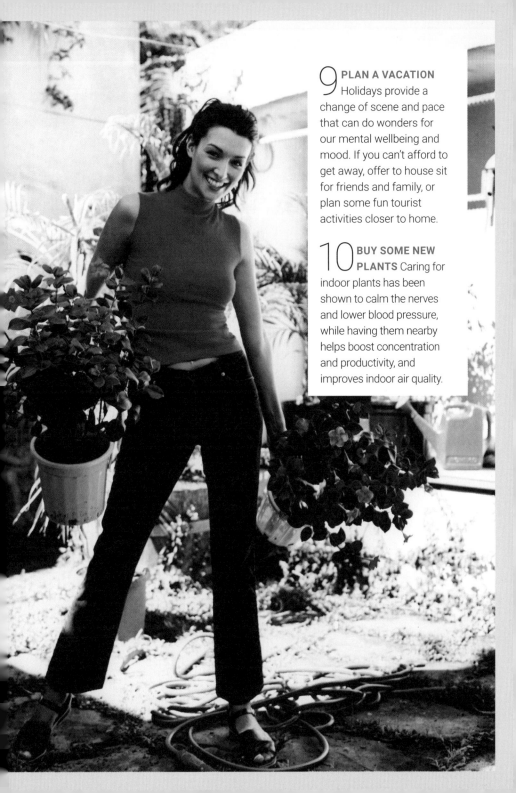

9 PLAN A VACATION Holidays provide a change of scene and pace that can do wonders for our mental wellbeing and mood. If you can't afford to get away, offer to house sit for friends and family, or plan some fun tourist activities closer to home.

10 BUY SOME NEW PLANTS Caring for indoor plants has been shown to calm the nerves and lower blood pressure, while having them nearby helps boost concentration and productivity, and improves indoor air quality.

DECEMBER						
S	M	T	W	T	F	S
31					1	2
3	4	5	6	7	8	9
10	11	12	13	14	15	16
17	18	19	20	21	22	23
24	25	26	27	28	29	30

JANUARY						
S	M	T	W	T	F	S
	1	2	3	4	5	6
7	8	9	10	11	12	13
14	15	16	17	18	19	20
21	22	23	24	25	26	27
28	29	30	31			

FEBRUARY						
S	M	T	W	T	F	S
				1	2	3
4	5	6	7	8	9	10
11	12	13	14	15	16	17
18	19	20	21	22	23	24
25	26	27	28	29		

1 MONDAY NEW YEAR'S DAY

2 TUESDAY

3 WEDNESDAY

4 THURSDAY

January
2024

5 FRIDAY

6 SATURDAY

FLEXIBILITY IS KEY when adopting a new routine. Implement one new habit at a time, and move things around to match your energy levels and daily commitments.

7 SUNDAY

DECEMBER

S	M	T	W	T	F	S
31					1	2
3	4	5	6	7	8	9
10	11	12	13	14	15	16
17	18	19	20	21	22	23
24	25	26	27	28	29	30

JANUARY

S	M	T	W	T	F	S
	1	2	3	4	5	6
7	8	9	10	11	12	13
14	15	16	17	18	19	20
21	22	23	24	25	26	27
28	29	30	31			

FEBRUARY

S	M	T	W	T	F	S
				1	2	3
4	5	6	7	8	9	10
11	12	13	14	15	16	17
18	19	20	21	22	23	24
25	26	27	28	29		

8 MONDAY

9 TUESDAY

10 WEDNESDAY

11 THURSDAY

12 FRIDAY

13 SATURDAY

14 SUNDAY

	DECEMBER					
S	M	T	W	T	F	S
31					1	2
3	4	5	6	7	8	9
10	11	12	13	14	15	16
17	18	19	20	21	22	23
24	25	26	27	28	29	30

	JANUARY					
S	M	T	W	T	F	S
	1	2	3	4	5	6
7	8	9	10	11	12	13
14	15	16	17	18	19	20
21	22	23	24	25	26	27
28	29	30	31			

	FEBRUARY					
S	M	T	W	T	F	S
				1	2	3
4	5	6	7	8	9	10
11	12	13	14	15	16	17
18	19	20	21	22	23	24
25	26	27	28	29		

15 MONDAY

16 TUESDAY

17 WEDNESDAY

18 THURSDAY

19 FRIDAY

20 SATURDAY

SWAP COFFEE FOR GREEN TEA. Packed with antioxidants, green tea may be linked with a decreased risk of heart disease and certain types of cancer.

21 SUNDAY

DECEMBER						
S	M	T	W	T	F	S
31					1	2
3	4	5	6	7	8	9
10	11	12	13	14	15	16
17	18	19	20	21	22	23
24	25	26	27	28	29	30

JANUARY						
S	M	T	W	T	F	S
	1	2	3	4	5	6
7	8	9	10	11	12	13
14	15	16	17	18	19	20
21	22	23	24	25	26	27
28	29	30	31			

FEBRUARY						
S	M	T	W	T	F	S
				1	2	3
4	5	6	7	8	9	10
11	12	13	14	15	16	17
18	19	20	21	22	23	24
25	26	27	28	29		

22 MONDAY

23 TUESDAY

24 WEDNESDAY

25 THURSDAY

26 FRIDAY AUSTRALIA DAY

27 SATURDAY

> **ADD A 10-MINUTE RUN TO YOUR DAILY WALK** to improve bone health. This is particularly important after menopause, when bone density loss increases.

28 SUNDAY

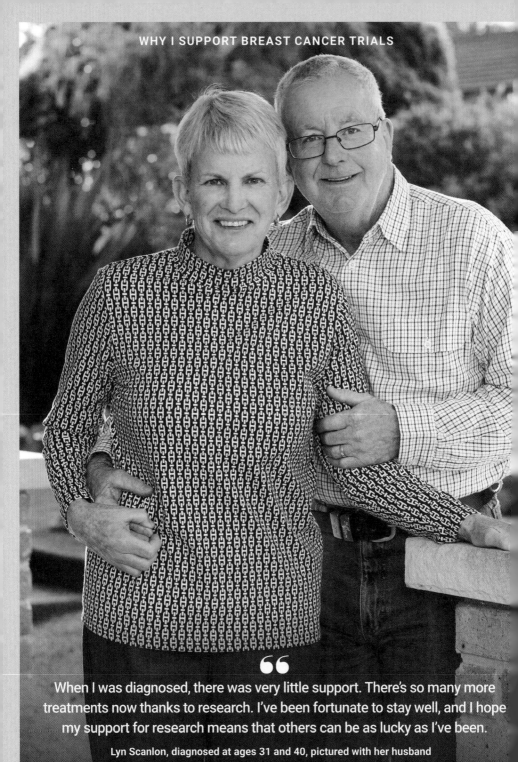

66

When I was diagnosed, there was very little support. There's so many more treatments now thanks to research. I've been fortunate to stay well, and I hope my support for research means that others can be as lucky as I've been.

Lyn Scanlon, diagnosed at ages 31 and 40, pictured with her husband

let's talk about
BEING ACTIVE

No matter how old you are, moving your body every day can have a positive impact on all areas of your health. Find ways to make physical activity a regular part of your lifestyle to reap the rewards.

While we understand the importance of getting our recommended 30 to 60 minutes of exercise each day (up to five hours per week), sometimes life, self-doubt or a little bit of self-sabotage gets in the way. Here are some of the most common exercise hurdles that women face, and how to overcome them.

Procrastination If you're new to exercise, it's easy to find excuses to put it off. The answer: just start. Any amount of exercise is better than none, so start small and see what your body and schedule can handle.

Lack of time Working, taking care of others and running a household can leave little free time for exercise. Talk to your family about ways they can help with tasks to free up your time. Also look for ways to build exercise into your lifestyle. Walk to the shops, do 10 squats in between activities or plan active outings with the kids.

Illness There are times when you shouldn't exercise while unwell – for example, if you're dizzy, dehydrated or have a chest infection. But it is possible to exercise if symptoms are mild. Keep it gentle and low-impact, such as a stroll around the block or some yoga stretches. If you have a chronic health condition, like cancer, arthritis or heart disease, speak to your doctor about appropriate forms of exercise.

Injury This is dependent on the type of injury, and should involve consulting your doctor or exercise physiologist about safe ways to exercise without jeopardising recovery. Ask yourself, "When I do this movement, do I feel better, worse or the same?" If you feel worse, seek guidance.

Boredom You won't like every type of exercise, and that's OK. Try different activities until you find one you do enjoy, or incorporate a mix of options. Why not enlist a friend to be active with you or join a group activity to make it more enjoyable.

Unrealistic expectations Setting an unachievable goal can quickly railroad good intentions. For example, attempting to drop a dress size in one week or signing up for a marathon when you've never been a runner. Instead, set realistic, adjustable and sustainable goals, such as doing 10 minutes on the exercise bike every day or going swimming twice a week.

For more information, visit Exercise & Sports Science Australia; exerciseright.com.au

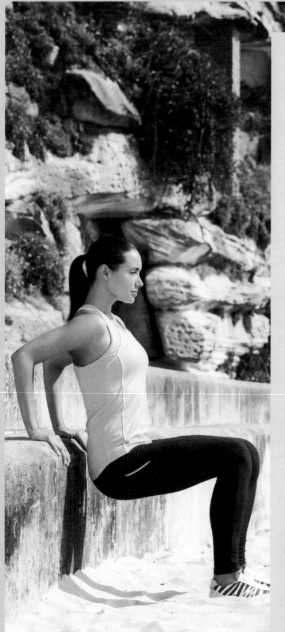

Budget-friendly ways to exercise

With the cost of living on an upwards trajectory, gym memberships or paid exercise classes are often one of the first things to be stripped from the budget. But there are still plenty of ways to exercise each day without placing a strain on your finances. Consider these options.

Go for a walk, run or bike ride

Look on YouTube for online exercise classes delivered by qualified experts

Use household equipment for weight training, such as a sturdy chair for tricep dips or bottles of water as weights

Go for a swim at a beach swimming pool

Use outdoor gym equipment at the park

Start a yoga club with your friends and take turns hosting

Search for unwanted gym equipment on Gumtree or Marketplace, or in council waste collections

Look on local community noticeboards for free Tai Chi groups, training sessions or dance workshops

Sign up for online fitness events, such as fun runs, charity walks or Zumba parties, where you challenge yourself to reach a goal and raise money for a worthwhile cause at the same time

Meet friends at the park for a game of soccer or netball

Check if your health fund or employer offers discounts on gym memberships or equipment.

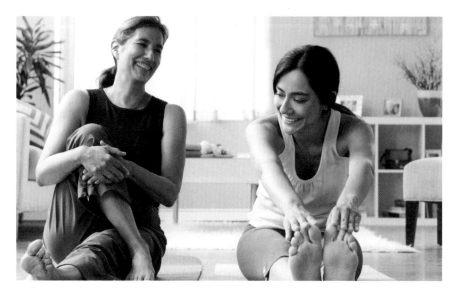

Exercise in your 60s and beyond

Moving our bodies every day becomes increasingly important as we get older. Exercise enhances strength and flexibility, which then helps with coordination and balance. Being physically active can also prevent weight gain and increase mobility. Exercising from a young age will benefit your physical health in the future, however, it's never too late to start moving. Studies show older women can achieve significant health benefits after just two or three months of regular exercise. Following the current guidelines, women over the age of 65 need at least 30 minutes of moderate intensity activity on most, if not all, days. In addition, aim to include exercises that focus on strength and flexibility three times a week. It sounds a lot, but you may be doing some of it already. Use this breakdown to tick all the boxes.

MODERATE INTENSITY ACTIVITIES CAN BE...	STRENGTH ACTIVITIES CAN BE...	FLEXIBILITY ACTIVITIES CAN BE...
Brisk walking	Weight training (including using your own body weight)	Tai Chi
Jogging	Resistance training	Yoga
Cycling	Gardening (digging, raking and lifting)	Pilates
Swimming	Climbing stairs	Dancing
Golf (without the cart)	Lifting and carrying (bags of groceries or young children)	Lawn bowls
Tennis	Stand up paddle boarding	Mopping or vacuuming
Aerobics		Stretching
Kayaking		
Dancing		
Mowing the lawn		
Heavy gardening		

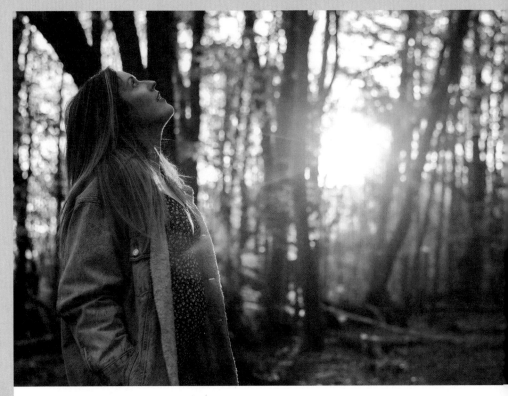

What is forest bathing?

Based on the Japanese practice of shinrin-yoku (meaning 'forest bath'), spending time in nature has been linked to reduced levels of stress and anxiety, better sleep quality and enhanced immunity. As well, it takes us away from the artificial lighting, screens and air-conditioning that we're constantly surrounded by indoors, which can place a strain on our mental and physical wellbeing.

Despite the name, it's not about taking a bath in the middle of a forest, but rather, finding a pocket of nature – be it a park, beach, garden or bush reserve – where you can switch off and enjoy the present moment. Just one 20-minute forest bathing session a month will do wonders for your stress levels. Here's how to get the most from your forest bathing experience.

1 **Stay local.** This reduces potential stressors of traffic or parking, and makes it easier to spend time in nature more often.

2 **Leave your phone behind** or switch it off. If you're walking with a friend, do so silently for at least five minutes.

3 **Walk slowly and mindfully**, savouring the sights, sounds and smells. You can increase the pace later, but starting slowly will give you the best benefits.

4 **Go barefoot if safe to do so**, or lie on a patch of grass, sand or a smooth rock to immerse yourself in your surroundings.

5 **You might like to meditate** or practise Tai Chi, build a sand castle or simply find a place to sit and be still.

6 **Don't focus on the destination.** Simply wander where you like, then head back the way you came when you're ready.

WE NEED YOUR FEEDBACK

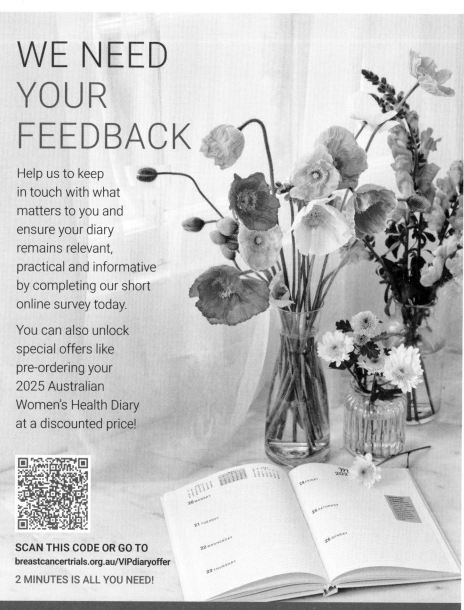

Help us to keep in touch with what matters to you and ensure your diary remains relevant, practical and informative by completing our short online survey today.

You can also unlock special offers like pre-ordering your 2025 Australian Women's Health Diary at a discounted price!

SCAN THIS CODE OR GO TO
breastcancertrials.org.au/VIPdiaryoffer

2 MINUTES IS ALL YOU NEED!

The Australian Women's Health Diary is an initiative of Breast Cancer Trials produced in conjunction with our friends at The Australian Women's Weekly. For 26 years, not only has this diary helped Australian women to be organised and informed about their health, it has also saved lives from breast cancer.

Learn more at breastcancertrials.org.au or call 1800 423 444.

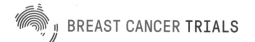 BREAST CANCER **TRIALS**

JANUARY

S	M	T	W	T	F	S
	1	2	3	4	5	6
7	8	9	10	11	12	13
14	15	16	17	18	19	20
21	22	23	24	25	26	27
28	29	30	31			

FEBRUARY

S	M	T	W	T	F	S
				1	2	3
4	5	6	7	8	9	10
11	12	13	14	15	16	17
18	19	20	21	22	23	24
25	26	27	28	29		

MARCH

S	M	T	W	T	F	S
31					1	2
3	4	5	6	7	8	9
10	11	12	13	14	15	16
17	18	19	20	21	22	23
24	25	26	27	28	29	30

29 MONDAY

30 TUESDAY

31 WEDNESDAY

1 THURSDAY

February
2024

2 FRIDAY

3 SATURDAY

ENSURE YOU'RE ADEQUATELY SUPPORTED during workouts by being professionally fitted for a sports bra and sneakers. Specify the type of exercise for tailored options.

4 SUNDAY

		JANUARY				
S	M	T	W	T	F	S
	1	2	3	4	5	6
7	8	9	10	11	12	13
14	15	16	17	18	19	20
21	22	23	24	25	26	27
28	29	30	31			

		FEBRUARY				
S	M	T	W	T	F	S
				1	2	3
4	5	6	7	8	9	10
11	12	13	14	15	16	17
18	19	20	21	22	23	24
25	26	27	28	29		

		MARCH				
S	M	T	W	T	F	S
31					1	2
3	4	5	6	7	8	9
10	11	12	13	14	15	16
17	18	19	20	21	22	23
24	25	26	27	28	29	30

5 MONDAY

6 TUESDAY

7 WEDNESDAY ISRA AND MI'RAJ (ISLAMIC HOLY DAY)

8 THURSDAY

9 FRIDAY

10 SATURDAY LUNAR NEW YEAR

HAVING A BABY?
Maintain physical activity to prepare your body for birth and assist its recovery. Walking, swimming, yoga and Pilates are good low-impact exercise options.

11 SUNDAY

	JANUARY								FEBRUARY								MARCH					
S	M	T	W	T	F	S		S	M	T	W	T	F	S		S	M	T	W	T	F	S
	1	2	3	4	5	6						1	2	3		31					1	2
7	8	9	10	11	12	13		4	5	6	7	8	9	10		3	4	5	6	7	8	9
14	15	16	17	18	19	20		11	12	13	14	15	16	17		10	11	12	13	14	15	16
21	22	23	24	25	26	27		18	19	20	21	22	23	24		17	18	19	20	21	22	23
28	29	30	31					25	26	27	28	29				24	25	26	27	28	29	30

12 MONDAY

13 TUESDAY

14 WEDNESDAY VALENTINE'S DAY

15 THURSDAY

16 FRIDAY

17 SATURDAY

KEEP AN EXERCISE DIARY to note down small but significant improvements, such as faster run times, better sleep, more energy or your clothes feeling less tight.

18 SUNDAY

JANUARY

S	M	T	W	T	F	S
		1	2	3	4	5	6
7	8	9	10	11	12	13
14	15	16	17	18	19	20
21	22	23	24	25	26	27
28	29	30	31			

FEBRUARY

S	M	T	W	T	F	S
					1	2	3
4	5	6	7	8	9	10
11	12	13	14	15	16	17
18	19	20	21	22	23	24
25	26	27	28	29		

MARCH

S	M	T	W	T	F	S
31					1	2
3	4	5	6	7	8	9
10	11	12	13	14	15	16
17	18	19	20	21	22	23
24	25	26	27	28	29	30

19 MONDAY

20 TUESDAY

21 WEDNESDAY

22 THURSDAY

February
2024

23 FRIDAY

24 SATURDAY

25 SUNDAY

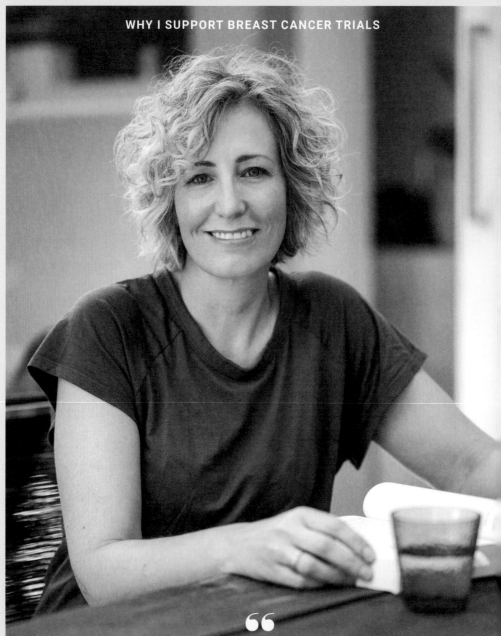

> My diagnosis turned my life upside down. But I have never once wondered 'why me?' Good people get cancer and it can feel a little bit like a lottery. I've made positive changes to my life and learned to appreciate the small kindnesses and small wins along the way. I try to live in hope, not fear.

Diane Barker, diagnosed at age 44

let's talk about
NUTRITION

The food we eat is our fuel for the day, and can have long-term effects on our health and wellbeing. With this in mind, set yourself on a nutritionally balanced path by making the very best choices.

While eating two serves of fruit and five serves of vegetables every day is the cornerstone of a healthy diet, aiming for a variety of colours will reap even more rewards. That's because fruit and vegetables fall into five colour categories, each with their own set of disease-fighting phytochemicals and health benefits.

Taste the rainbow

RED Tomatoes, strawberries and watermelon get their rosy blush from the natural plant pigment lycopene, which may help reduce the risk of cancer and boost heart health. They also have potassium to help protect against osteoporosis, and vitamin C for immune health.

BLUE/PURPLE Beetroot, blueberries, eggplant and plums get their colour from the pigment anthocyanin, which is thought to fight cell damage and help prevent cancer, stroke and heart disease. Manganese can also assist calcium absorption, blood sugar regulation and brain function.

ORANGE/YELLOW Carotenoids give this group their colour. One type of carotenoid, betacarotene, is found in carrot, pumpkin and sweet potato, and converts to vitamin A to promote eye and skin health. Lutein is another, found in corn, rockmelon and squash, and may help prevent vision loss.

GREEN Cruciferous greens like broccoli and cabbage have a host of cancer-fighting phytochemicals including carotenoids, indoles and glucosinolates. Leafy greens like spinach and broccoli also contain folate for healthy cell growth.

BROWN/WHITE Anthoxanthins in onions, cauliflower and mushrooms deliver antiviral and antioxidant benefits, and may help reduce the risk of stroke. Then there's the potassium in bananas and potatoes, which may help reduce high blood pressure.

HOW TO ADD MORE COLOUR TO YOUR DIET
- Incorporate two or three different-coloured fruit or vegetables at each meal.
- Enjoy snacks that centre around fruit and veg, such as carrot and cucumber sticks with dip, berries and yoghurt, grapes and cheese, or fruit kebabs.
- Grow your own fruit and vegetables, and try unusual variations of traditional favourites, like yellow tomatoes, purple beans or white eggplant.
- Encourage kids to track their colour choices on a chart using colour-coordinated stickers.

For more information, visit Nutrition Australia; nutritionaustralia.org

Nutrition myths debunked

The internet and social media are full of misleading information about what is deemed "healthy" or "good for you". Here, we debunk some of the more common nutrition mistruths to help you make informed decisions about what you eat.

MYTH: Low-fat is best

When it comes to fat in our diet, quality overrules quantity. Saturated fats in processed meats, pastries, cakes and biscuits should be limited, however, small amounts of good fats like avocado, olive oil, nuts, seeds and oily fish provide us with essential fatty acids and can help protect against heart disease. Foods labelled as low-fat often contain added sugar or salt to improve their taste, so aren't always better than unaltered, higher-fat alternatives.

MYTH: Carbs make you fat

While eating too much can lead to weight gain, many carbohydrates deliver a host of benefits. Complex carbohydrates like wholegrain bread, pasta, cereals and brown rice, fruit, vegetables, legumes, milk and dairy give us energy, keep us full, provide fibre for digestive health and can help prevent blood sugar spikes. Aim for six serves of grains per day until age 50, then three to four serves thereafter.

MYTH: Eating meat builds muscle

It's true that protein contains amino acids for muscle building and recovery, however, plant proteins like soy, quinoa, buckwheat, nuts and legumes will provide the same benefits if you eat a variety of plant foods from different plant sources throughout the day. Women need 2.5 serves of meat, poultry, fish or non-meat sources each day.

MYTH: Sugar is evil

Too much refined sugar, found in soft drink, cakes, biscuits, chocolate bars and lollies, can cause fluctuating energy levels, interrupted sleep, skin inflammation, mood swings, tooth decay and increased heart disease risk. But natural sugars in fruit, vegetables, milk and natural yoghurt do not – in fact, they offer other nutritional benefits like fibre, protein and calcium.

MYTH: Red wine is good for the heart

Research shows that drinking any form of alcohol can increase the risk of many types of cancer. In the past, red wine was hailed as the best choice due to its antioxidant content, however, the current advice is to get your antioxidants from fruit and vegetable sources and reduce your alcohol intake – no more than 10 standard drinks a week, or no more than four standard drinks per day.

MYTH: Drinking juice is the best way to get your five serves of veg and two serves of fruit per day

Juicing breaks down the beneficial fibre found in the skin and pectin of fruit and vegetables, while pre-bottled juices are often laden with sugar. Instead, eat your fruit and vegetables in their whole forms to gain the full benefits.

MYTH: Healthy eating is expensive

There are lots of ways to eat well without breaking the budget. Shop seasonally for fruit and vegetables or grow your own; buy staples like wholemeal pasta, brown rice, oats and dried legumes in bulk; and look to frozen fruit and vegetables and long-life milk to prevent food waste.

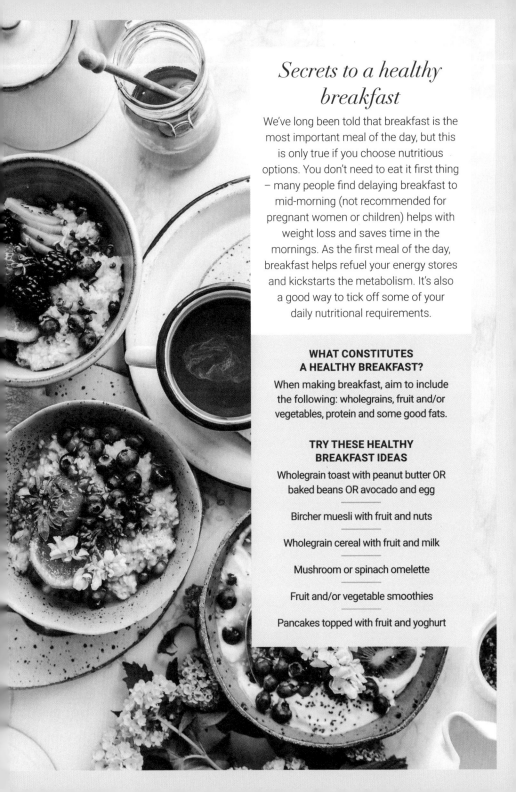

Secrets to a healthy breakfast

We've long been told that breakfast is the most important meal of the day, but this is only true if you choose nutritious options. You don't need to eat it first thing – many people find delaying breakfast to mid-morning (not recommended for pregnant women or children) helps with weight loss and saves time in the mornings. As the first meal of the day, breakfast helps refuel your energy stores and kickstarts the metabolism. It's also a good way to tick off some of your daily nutritional requirements.

WHAT CONSTITUTES A HEALTHY BREAKFAST?

When making breakfast, aim to include the following: wholegrains, fruit and/or vegetables, protein and some good fats.

TRY THESE HEALTHY BREAKFAST IDEAS

Wholegrain toast with peanut butter OR baked beans OR avocado and egg

Bircher muesli with fruit and nuts

Wholegrain cereal with fruit and milk

Mushroom or spinach omelette

Fruit and/or vegetable smoothies

Pancakes topped with fruit and yoghurt

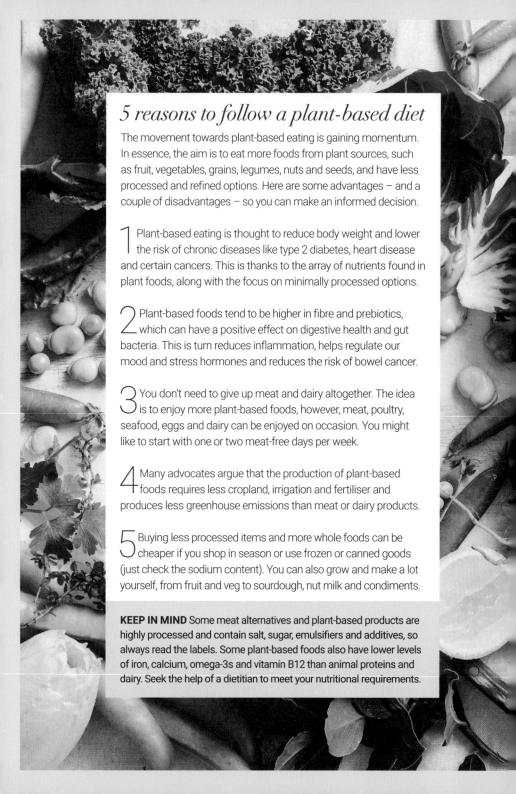

5 reasons to follow a plant-based diet

The movement towards plant-based eating is gaining momentum. In essence, the aim is to eat more foods from plant sources, such as fruit, vegetables, grains, legumes, nuts and seeds, and have less processed and refined options. Here are some advantages – and a couple of disadvantages – so you can make an informed decision.

1 Plant-based eating is thought to reduce body weight and lower the risk of chronic diseases like type 2 diabetes, heart disease and certain cancers. This is thanks to the array of nutrients found in plant foods, along with the focus on minimally processed options.

2 Plant-based foods tend to be higher in fibre and prebiotics, which can have a positive effect on digestive health and gut bacteria. This is turn reduces inflammation, helps regulate our mood and stress hormones and reduces the risk of bowel cancer.

3 You don't need to give up meat and dairy altogether. The idea is to enjoy more plant-based foods, however, meat, poultry, seafood, eggs and dairy can be enjoyed on occasion. You might like to start with one or two meat-free days per week.

4 Many advocates argue that the production of plant-based foods requires less cropland, irrigation and fertiliser and produces less greenhouse emissions than meat or dairy products.

5 Buying less processed items and more whole foods can be cheaper if you shop in season or use frozen or canned goods (just check the sodium content). You can also grow and make a lot yourself, from fruit and veg to sourdough, nut milk and condiments.

KEEP IN MIND Some meat alternatives and plant-based products are highly processed and contain salt, sugar, emulsifiers and additives, so always read the labels. Some plant-based foods also have lower levels of iron, calcium, omega-3s and vitamin B12 than animal proteins and dairy. Seek the help of a dietitian to meet your nutritional requirements.

Practising portion control

Research suggests that two-thirds of Australian adults are overweight or obese due to poor dietary choices. In many cases, our serving sizes, or portions, play a large part in these statistics, and the reasons for this can vary.

For instance, many of us were raised to finish everything on our plates, and we carry this habit into adulthood. Other factors like sleep deprivation, eating on the run, hormonal fluctuations and some medications can cause us to make unhealthy food choices as well as interfere with our ability to tune into our body's fullness cues. The ability to detect fullness often reduces with age, and, along with other factors like menopause and lack of exercise, can contribute to "middle-aged spread". In addition, portion sizes of discretionary foods like burgers, chips and pizza have grown over the years, adding unwanted kilojoules to our daily intake.

So how can we bring our portion sizes back in line with a healthy range? Ultimately, we need to slow down when we eat and become more intuitive eaters. Try to differentiate between the various stages of hunger – peckish, hungry or ravenous, and satisfied, full or uncomfortably full – and eat slowly and mindfully to determine which stage you're at. Minimise distractions, and put down your cutlery between mouthfuls to properly chew, taste and swallow every bite. Check in with yourself at regular intervals and aim to stop eating once you feel satisfied and comfortably full.

If you find mindful eating difficult, you can also structure your meals using the plate model, which involves dividing your plate as follows:

1 Approximately ½ of the plate with mostly non-starchy vegetables and a little fruit.

2 Roughly ¼ of the plate for starchy vegetables, grains and complex carbohydrates, such as wholegrain pasta, rice, cereals and noodles.

3 About ¼ of the plate reserved for protein, be it lean red meat, poultry, seafood, eggs, legumes, tofu or dairy.

4 A small slice of the plate for good fats, like nuts, seeds, avocado and extra virgin olive oil.

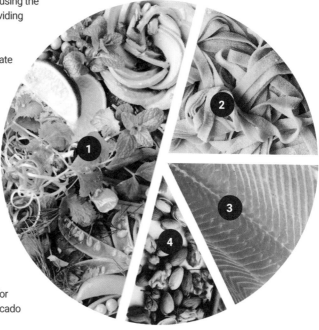

FEBRUARY						
S	M	T	W	T	F	S
				1	2	3
4	5	6	7	8	9	10
11	12	13	14	15	16	17
18	19	20	21	22	23	24
25	26	27	28	29		

MARCH						
S	M	T	W	T	F	S
31					1	2
3	4	5	6	7	8	9
10	11	12	13	14	15	16
17	18	19	20	21	22	23
24	25	26	27	28	29	30

APRIL						
S	M	T	W	T	F	S
	1	2	3	4	5	6
7	8	9	10	11	12	13
14	15	16	17	18	19	20
21	22	23	24	25	26	27
28	29	30				

26 MONDAY

27 TUESDAY

28 WEDNESDAY

29 THURSDAY

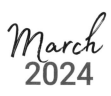

March
2024

1 FRIDAY

2 SATURDAY

KEEN TO CURB YOUR CAFFEINE INTAKE? Cut back gradually to lessen any withdrawal symptoms by eliminating one cup of coffee or can of cola every few days.

3 SUNDAY

FEBRUARY

S	M	T	W	T	F	S
				1	2	3
4	5	6	7	8	9	10
11	12	13	14	15	16	17
18	19	20	21	22	23	24
25	26	27	28	29		

MARCH

S	M	T	W	T	F	S
31					1	2
3	4	5	6	7	8	9
10	11	12	13	14	15	16
17	18	19	20	21	22	23
24	25	26	27	28	29	30

APRIL

S	M	T	W	T	F	S
	1	2	3	4	5	6
7	8	9	10	11	12	13
14	15	16	17	18	19	20
21	22	23	24	25	26	27
28	29	30				

4 MONDAY LABOUR DAY (WA)

5 TUESDAY

6 WEDNESDAY

7 THURSDAY

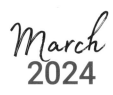

March
2024

8 FRIDAY INTERNATIONAL WOMEN'S DAY

9 SATURDAY

**SWITCHING
TO A MILK
ALTERNATIVE**
like soy, almond,
oat or rice milk?
Make sure you
pick a product with
no added sugar
and a calcium
content of 100mg
per 100ml.

10 SUNDAY

FEBRUARY						
S	M	T	W	T	F	S
					1	2	3
4	5	6	7	8	9	10
11	12	13	14	15	16	17
18	19	20	21	22	23	24
25	26	27	28	29		

MARCH						
S	M	T	W	T	F	S
31					1	2
3	4	5	6	7	8	9
10	11	12	13	14	15	16
17	18	19	20	21	22	23
24	25	26	27	28	29	30

APRIL						
S	M	T	W	T	F	S
	1	2	3	4	5	6
7	8	9	10	11	12	13
14	15	16	17	18	19	20
21	22	23	24	25	26	27
28	29	30				

11 MONDAY
LABOUR DAY (VIC), EIGHT HOURS DAY (TAS), ADELAIDE CUP (SA), CANBERRA DAY (ACT), RAMADAN STARTS

12 TUESDAY

13 WEDNESDAY

14 THURSDAY

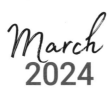

March
2024

15 FRIDAY

16 SATURDAY

17 SUNDAY ST PATRICK'S DAY

F E B R U A R Y						
S	M	T	W	T	F	S
				1	2	3
4	5	6	7	8	9	10
11	12	13	14	15	16	17
18	19	20	21	22	23	24
25	26	27	28	29		

M A R C H						
S	M	T	W	T	F	S
31					1	2
3	4	5	6	7	8	9
10	11	12	13	14	15	16
17	18	19	20	21	22	23
24	25	26	27	28	29	30

A P R I L						
S	M	T	W	T	F	S
	1	2	3	4	5	6
7	8	9	10	11	12	13
14	15	16	17	18	19	20
21	22	23	24	25	26	27
28	29	30				

18 MONDAY

19 TUESDAY

20 WEDNESDAY NOWRUZ (PERSIAN NEW YEAR)

21 THURSDAY HARMONY DAY, NATIONAL CLOSE THE GAP DAY

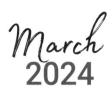

March
2024

22 FRIDAY

23 SATURDAY

> **MINIMISE YOUR INTAKE OF SUGARY FOODS** like soft drink, lollies, fruit juice, sports drinks, cakes and biscuits to help prevent weight gain, heart disease, acne and depression.

24 SUNDAY

FEBRUARY
S	M	T	W	T	F	S
				1	2	3
4	5	6	7	8	9	10
11	12	13	14	15	16	17
18	19	20	21	22	23	24
25	26	27	28	29		

MARCH
S	M	T	W	T	F	S
31					1	2
3	4	5	6	7	8	9
10	11	12	13	14	15	16
17	18	19	20	21	22	23
24	25	26	27	28	29	30

APRIL
S	M	T	W	T	F	S
	1	2	3	4	5	6
7	8	9	10	11	12	13
14	15	16	17	18	19	20
21	22	23	24	25	26	27
28	29	30				

25 MONDAY

26 TUESDAY

27 WEDNESDAY

28 THURSDAY

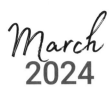

March
2024

29 FRIDAY GOOD FRIDAY

30 SATURDAY

> **DRINK SIX TO EIGHT GLASSES OF WATER** each day to help manage appetite, replenish energy levels and remove toxins from your body and skin.

31 SUNDAY EASTER SUNDAY

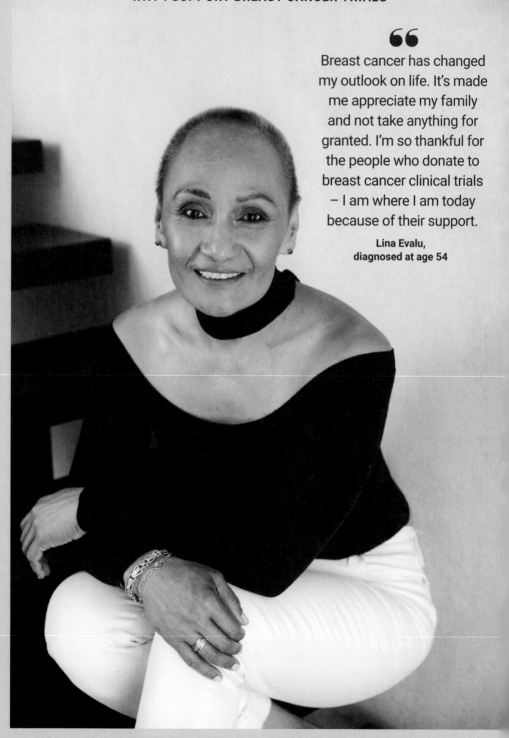

"

Breast cancer has changed my outlook on life. It's made me appreciate my family and not take anything for granted. I'm so thankful for the people who donate to breast cancer clinical trials – I am where I am today because of their support.

**Lina Evalu,
diagnosed at age 54**

let's talk about
WOMEN'S HEALTH

There are a number of health concerns and topics that affect women specifically, due to our gynaecological makeup and societal attitudes. In many cases, knowledge is the best form of prevention and protection.

Domestic violence and abuse is a growing concern in Australia, with a surge of instances reported following the 2020 and 2021 Covid-19 lockdowns. One in four women have experienced emotional abuse by a current or previous partner, placing them at higher risk of a range of mental health conditions, such as post-traumatic stress disorder (PTSD), depression, anxiety, substance abuse and thoughts of suicide. Violence against women can take many forms, such as physical, sexual, social, emotional and financial abuse, as well as controlling, coercive and intimidating behaviour, and it occurs across all cultures and communities. It's important to know the signs of an unhealthy relationship and where to seek help, should you need it.

What is a healthy relationship?
In a healthy relationship, you have the freedom to see family and friends on your own, have your own hobbies and interests and can make your own decisions. You and your partner communicate with each other respectfully and feel comfortable expressing your feelings. Above all else, your relationship should bring more happiness than sadness or stress, and you should always feel safe.

When relationships turn toxic
Most relationships go through ups and downs, and you and your partner might have disagreements or periods of unhappiness. Abuse, on the other hand, is a pattern of behaviour that stems from a desire to hold power over someone. An abusive partner might threaten or put you down, prevent you from seeing friends and family, take control of your finances, act jealous or resentful towards you or deliberately hurt you. You might also notice changes in yourself, such as feeling constantly on edge around your partner, not feeling like you have a voice, withdrawing from activities you once loved or neglecting your health and self-care.

Where to get support
In some instances, if you and your partner can acknowledge that your relationship is struggling and are both willing to work on it, individual or couples counselling is a great first step. However, if you are worried about unhealthy, abusive or violent behaviour in any of your relationships, you can contact online counselling service 1800RESPECT using the details below for confidential advice and support. Reach out to friends and family, and if you are in danger, please call Triple Zero (000) immediately.

For more information, visit 1800RESPECT; 1800respect.org.au.

Contraception after 40

As you get older and your hormones and health risk factors shift, you may want to reconsider your contraceptive methods. The two main roles of contraception are to prevent pregnancy and to protect against sexually transmitted infections (STIs). As you get older, your fertility decreases and being in a committed relationship reduces (but doesn't eliminate) the possibility of contracting an STI. This makes emergency contraceptive options like condoms and the morning after pill less necessary (unless you're just starting a new relationship), and set-and-forget forms of birth control or permanent solutions more appealing. Use this table to weigh up your options, bearing in mind that some form of contraception is recommended until at least one or two years after menopause (one year after your last period).

CONTRACEPTIVE	HOW IT WORKS
Combined oral contraceptive pill (the Pill)	Two hormones – oestrogen and progesterone – combine to stop the ovaries from releasing an egg each month. They also thicken the mucus at the entrance of the cervix to prevent sperm from entering the womb.
Progestogen-only pill (the mini pill)	Containing a very small dose of progestogen, the mini pill thickens the mucus in the cervix to prevent sperm from entering.
Mirena progestogen	Inserted into the uterus through the vagina (with or without anaesthetic), the Mirena contains a slow-release progestogen to suppress ovulation, thicken the cervical mucus and prevent egg fertilisation.
Copper intra-uterine device (IUD)	Inserted like the Mirena, the IUD is toxic to sperm and also stops a fertilised egg from settling into the uterus.
Progestogen implants (Implanon)	The matchstick-sized plastic rod is inserted under the skin of the inner upper arm under local anaesthetic. Containing etonogestrel, it stops the production and release of eggs and thickens the cervical mucus.
Contraceptive hormonal vaginal ring	A small, pliable ring containing oestrogen and progestogen is inserted into the vagina for three weeks to stop the ovaries from releasing an egg.
Fertility tracking	Tracking a woman's cycle using apps and basal temperature measurements can help pinpoint when ovulation occurs as well as her "fertile window", which can last from five days pre-ovulation to five days post-ovulation.
Tubal ligation (tubes tied)	Performed under general anaesthetic, this keyhole surgery involves having the woman's fallopian tubes clipped, cut and tied or sealed shut to prevent eggs travelling from the ovaries to the uterus.
Vasectomy	An option for men, a vasectomy is a minor procedure performed under general or local anaesthetic to sever and seal the tubes that carry sperm to the penis.

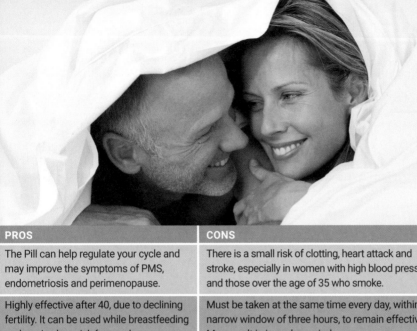

PROS	CONS
The Pill can help regulate your cycle and may improve the symptoms of PMS, endometriosis and perimenopause.	There is a small risk of clotting, heart attack and stroke, especially in women with high blood pressure, and those over the age of 35 who smoke.
Highly effective after 40, due to declining fertility. It can be used while breastfeeding and carries less risk for smokers.	Must be taken at the same time every day, within a narrow window of three hours, to remain effective. May result in irregular periods.
It can last five to seven years and is easily removed. Women often experience less menstrual blood loss and discomfort.	A small number of women may experience irregular spotting and bleeding or progestogen-related side effects like bloating, sore breasts and weight gain.
A medium-term, non-hormonal option that can last 5-10 years, or longer after age 40.	Some women may experience heavier and more painful bleeding.
An inexpensive option, Implanon lasts for three years.	Women may experience acne, breast tenderness and mood changes, and in some cases, menstrual irregularities that require the implant to be removed.
There may be less hormonal side effects than the Pill.	The same as the Pill, and additionally, it does not prevent against STIs.
A quick, simple method of contraception that doesn't require the use of medication.	There's a risk of pregnancy if not vigilant with tracking and accuracy. Another form of contraception is needed during the fertile window. No protection from STIs.
Many women choose this 99 per cent effective option if they are finished having children and no longer want to rely on contraceptives.	This permanent procedure cannot be reversed if you change your mind, and comes with a small risk of injury to the blood vessels, ureters and bowel, and a small risk of ectopic pregnancy. It does not protect against STIs.
Most men experience a quick recovery time. This method takes the pressure off the woman, who often carries the responsibility of using birth control.	A small risk of injury to the testicles. Not immediately effective, it requires a semen analysis at three months. While vasectomies can be reversed, it is not always successful. Does not protect against STIs.

For more information, visit Jean Hailes for Women's Health; jeanhailes.org.au

Spotlight on ovarian cancer

THE STATS Ovarian cancer is the most lethal gynaecological cancer in Australia, with approximately 1815 women diagnosed each year. Women over 50 have a higher risk of ovarian cancer, however younger women can also be diagnosed. With no screening tools available, many cases will have spread beyond the ovaries by the time they're found.

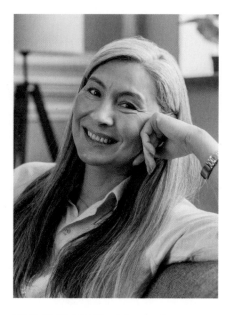

SYMPTOMS Many ovarian cancer symptoms can be vague and easily attributed to other conditions. The most common symptoms are:
- Abdominal bloating
- Back, abdominal or pelvic pain
- Feeling full after only eating a small amount
- Frequent or urgent urination
- Changes in bowel habits; constipation or diarrhoea
- Unexplained weight gain or loss
- Excessive fatigue
- Lower back pain
- Indigestion or nausea
- Bleeding after menopause or in between periods
- Pain during sex or bleeding after.

While many of these symptoms may not seem serious, it's always best to see your doctor.

RISK FACTORS The following factors may increase a woman's risk:
- Getting older (risk increases after age 50)
- A family history of ovarian, breast or bowel cancer
- Inheriting a BRCA1 or BRCA2 gene mutation
- Being of Ashkenazi Jewish descent
- Early onset of periods (before 12 years) or late menopause (55 and over)
- Having endometriosis
- Having diabetes
- Use of hormone replacement therapy (HRT)
- Being overweight
- Smoking
- Not having children, or having your first child after age 35.

DIAGNOSIS AND TREATMENT If you present with symptoms, your GP may perform a physical examination, order blood tests or send you for a transvaginal ultrasound, CT scan, PET scan or colonoscopy to check for abnormalities. A biopsy will then confirm a cancer diagnosis. Surgery is the main course of treatment, in conjunction with chemotherapy before or after surgery.

For more information, visit Ovarian Cancer Australia; ovariancancer.net.au

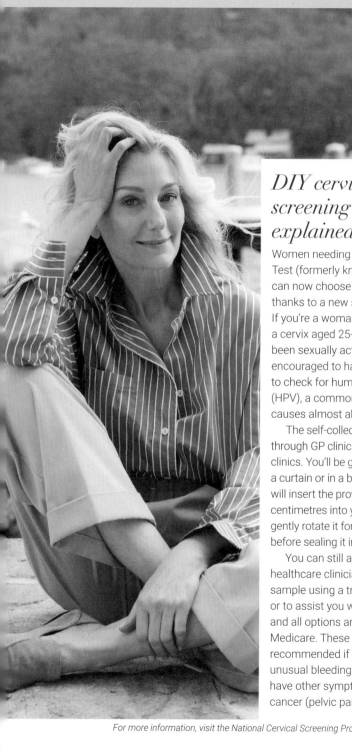

DIY cervical screening kits explained

Women needing a Cervical Screening Test (formerly known as a Pap smear) can now choose to do it themselves, thanks to a new self-collect option. If you're a woman or person with a cervix aged 25-74 and have ever been sexually active, you're encouraged to have a five-yearly test to check for human papillomavirus (HPV), a common infection that causes almost all cervical cancers.

The self-collection test is available through GP clinics and women's health clinics. You'll be given privacy behind a curtain or in a bathroom, where you will insert the provided swab a few centimetres into your vagina and gently rotate it for 20 to 30 seconds before sealing it in the provided bag.

You can still ask your GP or healthcare clinician to collect the sample using a traditional speculum or to assist you with self-collection, and all options are free under Medicare. These tests are not recommended if you're experiencing unusual bleeding, pain or discharge or have other symptoms of cervical cancer (pelvic pain, pain during sex).

For more information, visit the National Cervical Screening Program; health.gov.au/ncsp

		MARCH				
S	M	T	W	T	F	S
31					1	2
3	4	5	6	7	8	9
10	11	12	13	14	15	16
17	18	19	20	21	22	23
24	25	26	27	28	29	30

		APRIL				
S	M	T	W	T	F	S
	1	2	3	4	5	6
7	8	9	10	11	12	13
14	15	16	17	18	19	20
21	22	23	24	25	26	27
28	29	30				

		MAY				
S	M	T	W	T	F	S
			1	2	3	4
5	6	7	8	9	10	11
12	13	14	15	16	17	18
19	20	21	22	23	24	25
26	27	28	29	30	31	

1 MONDAY EASTER MONDAY

2 TUESDAY EASTER TUESDAY (TAS)

3 WEDNESDAY

4 THURSDAY

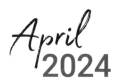

April 2024

5 FRIDAY

6 SATURDAY

7 SUNDAY DAYLIGHT SAVING TIME ENDS (ACT, NSW, SA, TAS, VIC)

S	M	T	W	T	F	S
		MARCH				
31					1	2
3	4	5	6	7	8	9
10	11	12	13	14	15	16
17	18	19	20	21	22	23
24	25	26	27	28	29	30

S	M	T	W	T	F	S
		APRIL				
	1	2	3	4	5	6
7	8	9	10	11	12	13
14	15	16	17	18	19	20
21	22	23	24	25	26	27
28	29	30				

S	M	T	W	T	F	S
		MAY				
			1	2	3	4
5	6	7	8	9	10	11
12	13	14	15	16	17	18
19	20	21	22	23	24	25
26	27	28	29	30	31	

8 MONDAY

9 TUESDAY

10 WEDNESDAY EID AL-FITR (ISLAMIC HOLIDAY)

11 THURSDAY

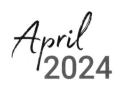

April
2024

12 FRIDAY

13 SATURDAY

14 SUNDAY

MARCH						
S	M	T	W	T	F	S
31					1	2
3	4	5	6	7	8	9
10	11	12	13	14	15	16
17	18	19	20	21	22	23
24	25	26	27	28	29	30

APRIL						
S	M	T	W	T	F	S
	1	2	3	4	5	6
7	8	9	10	11	12	13
14	15	16	17	18	19	20
21	22	23	24	25	26	27
28	29	30				

MAY						
S	M	T	W	T	F	S
			1	2	3	4
5	6	7	8	9	10	11
12	13	14	15	16	17	18
19	20	21	22	23	24	25
26	27	28	29	30	31	

15 MONDAY

16 TUESDAY

17 WEDNESDAY

18 THURSDAY

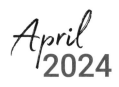

April
2024

19 FRIDAY

20 SATURDAY

21 SUNDAY

		MARCH							APRIL							MAY			
S	M	T	W	T	F	S	S	M	T	W	T	F	S	S	M	T	W	T	F	S
31					1	2		1	2	3	4	5	6				1	2	3	4
3	4	5	6	7	8	9	7	8	9	10	11	12	13	5	6	7	8	9	10	11
10	11	12	13	14	15	16	14	15	16	17	18	19	20	12	13	14	15	16	17	18
17	18	19	20	21	22	23	21	22	23	24	25	26	27	19	20	21	22	23	24	25
24	25	26	27	28	29	30	28	29	30					26	27	28	29	30	31	

22 MONDAY

23 TUESDAY PASSOVER BEGINS

24 WEDNESDAY

25 THURSDAY ANZAC DAY

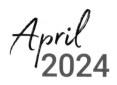

April
2024

26 FRIDAY

27 SATURDAY

28 SUNDAY

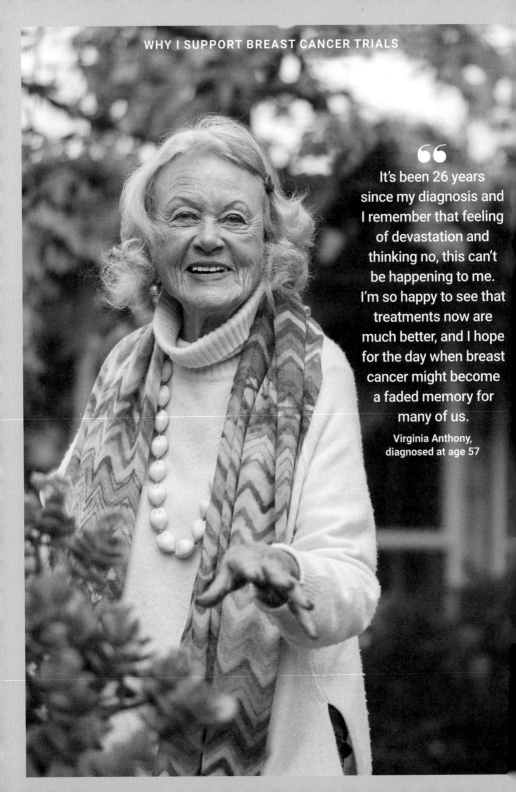

66

It's been 26 years since my diagnosis and I remember that feeling of devastation and thinking no, this can't be happening to me. I'm so happy to see that treatments now are much better, and I hope for the day when breast cancer might become a faded memory for many of us.

Virginia Anthony,
diagnosed at age 57

let's talk about
HEART HEALTH

Despite 20 Australian women losing their lives to heart disease each day, we often neglect our heart health. Correct this discrepancy by learning the risk factors of heart disease and making healthy lifestyle choices.

There's a misconception that heart disease only affects overweight, middle-aged men, but women are also susceptible. Reduce your risk by rectifying these common causes.

PHYSICAL INACTIVITY Sitting for long periods can cause weight gain, high blood pressure and high cholesterol, almost doubling the risk of coronary heart disease. **Help your heart** Start with a daily walk – it doesn't have to be 10,000 steps. From there, try other types of exercise, aiming for 30-60 minutes, five days a week.

POOR DIET Too many fatty, salty, overly processed foods can lead to obesity, high blood pressure, high cholesterol and diabetes. Drinking alcohol could also increase your risk of heart disease and stroke. **Help your heart** Eat a varied diet rich in fruit, vegetables, wholegrains, lean protein, legumes, nuts, seeds, reduced-fat dairy and healthy fats and oils. Stick to the national alcohol guidelines of no more than four standard drinks in one day and no more than 10 standard drinks per week.

SMOKING Accounting for one-fifth of all heart disease deaths, smoking causes plaque to build up inside the heart arteries, which can reduce blood flow and lead to a heart attack. The risk is higher if you smoke and take the oral contraceptive pill. **Help your heart** Quit today by calling 13 QUIT (137 848) or visit quit.org.au.

DEPRESSION & LONELINESS Stress and depression can cause your heart rate and blood pressure to rise. Similarly, feeling alone or isolated can increase our risk of a heart attack by 29 per cent. **Help your heart** Prioritise catch-ups with friends or seek support from a counsellor. Regular exercise can also boost the feel-good chemicals in your brain.

NON-MODIFIABLE FACTORS
Some genetic risk factors can't be eliminated, but should be flagged with your GP for monitoring. These include:
- a family history of heart disease and heart attack, particularly in female relatives before the age of 60 and male relatives before age 55
- diabetes
- pregnancy complications (such as preeclampsia, gestational diabetes or premature birth)
- reaching menopause
- being of Aboriginal or Torres Strait Islander descent.

For more information, visit the Victor Chang Cardiac Research Institute; victorchang.edu.au

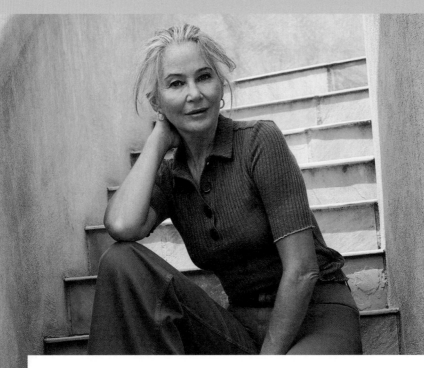

The signs of heart attack and stroke

For most women, the warning signs of heart attack or stroke can be subtle, and often go ignored. If you or someone you know experiences one or a combination of any of the following symptons, call Triple Zero (000) for immediate medical attention.

HEART ATTACK

- **Pressure or tightness in the chest**
- **Pain, discomfort or tightness in the jaw neck, shoulder, upper back or abdomen**
- **Shortness of breath with or without chest discomfort**
- **Pain in one or both arms**
- **Nausea, vomiting or indigestion**
- **Hot or cold sweats**
- **Light-headedness, dizziness or unusual feelings of fatigue**
- **Heart palpitations in combination with any of the above symptoms**

STROKE

- **Paralysis, weakness or numbness of the face, arms, legs or on one or both sides of the body**
- **Facial droop on one or both sides affecting the mouth and/or eyes**
- **Trouble speaking, particularly slurring or garbled speech**
- **Loss of vision, sudden blurring or decreased vision in one or both eyes**
- **Sudden and severe headache**
- **Vomiting, dizziness, loss of balance**
- **Difficulty swallowing**

What is angina?

Coronary heart disease (CHD), the most common form of heart disease, typically presents in one of two ways: as angina or as a heart attack. The symptoms of angina are similar to those of a heart attack: pain, heaviness or discomfort in the chest, arms, jaw, back or stomach, and in some cases, shortness of breath. But the main difference is that the symptoms of angina are temporary, often come on with physical activity or emotional upset, and usually go away after 10 or less minutes of rest.

Both angina and heart attack are most commonly caused by plaque build-up in the artery walls. In the case of angina, blood flow to the heart is reduced for a short period of time, while in a heart attack, blood flow is restricted entirely. If in doubt, always seek medical attention, as early intervention is crucial in the event of a heart attack.

If angina is diagnosed, your doctor can treat and manage it with medication, or in some cases, with surgery. You can also help reduce its effects by addressing any contributing lifestyle factors, such as lack of exercise, poor diet or smoking.

If the symptoms of your angina change, become unpredictable, last longer than usual or don't respond to rest or angina medications, call your doctor immediately or ring Triple Zero (000).

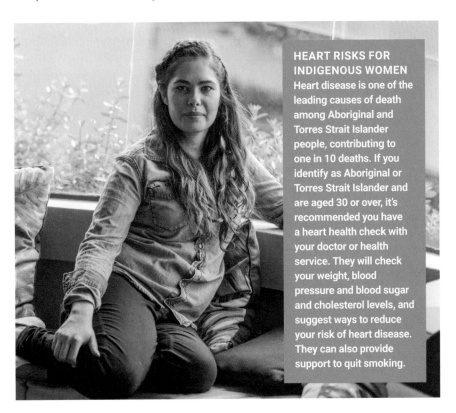

HEART RISKS FOR INDIGENOUS WOMEN
Heart disease is one of the leading causes of death among Aboriginal and Torres Strait Islander people, contributing to one in 10 deaths. If you identify as Aboriginal or Torres Strait Islander and are aged 30 or over, it's recommended you have a heart health check with your doctor or health service. They will check your weight, blood pressure and blood sugar and cholesterol levels, and suggest ways to reduce your risk of heart disease. They can also provide support to quit smoking.

9 legume-loaded recipes for heart health

Cheap, versatile and with a long shelf life, legumes have many health benefits, including helping to lower cholesterol and blood pressure – two leading causes of heart disease. Legumes take many forms, from chickpeas and lentils to kidney beans, peanuts and peas. Try these delicious ideas, introducing one type of legume at a time to avoid tummy upsets.

BREAKFAST

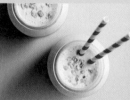 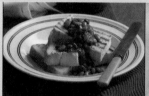 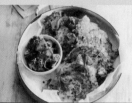

PB SMOOTHIE Add one tablespoon of peanut butter to a banana or berry smoothie for an extra dose of dietary fibre.

BEANS ON TOAST Make a low-salt alternative to baked beans using white beans, tomatoes, onion, garlic and paprika.

CORN & ZUCCHINI FRITTERS Use any fritter recipe, swapping white flour for chickpea flour for extra legume content.

LUNCH

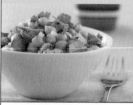 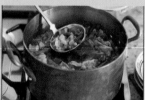 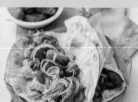

TUNA CHICKPEA SALAD Combine canned tuna and chickpeas with diced cucumber, avocado, corn and fresh parsley.

MINESTRONE Use a dried soup mix to make this legume-laden soup. Add stock, tomatoes, pasta and any chopped veg you have.

FALAFEL WRAP Combine canned chickpeas, onion, garlic, cumin, parsley and coriander in a food processor, roll and bake.

DINNER

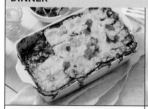 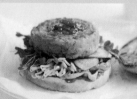 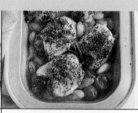

MEXICAN LASAGNE Try a twist on lasagne using capsicum, eggplant, corn, kidney beans and taco seasoning. Mince optional.

LENTIL & BEAN BURGERS Make patties by blending together soaked lentils, canned four bean mix, egg, onion and breadcrumbs.

CHICKEN CASSEROLE Brown chicken thighs on the stove. Add to a pan with cannellini beans, tomatoes and herbs and oven bake.

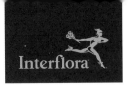

Make every moment brighter

Interflora is synonymous the world over with the feelings and sentiments that only flowers can evoke.

We make a good moment great, bad ones a little lighter and everyday moments a reason to be thankful. From expressions of love, to celebrations of success; from shared sorrows, to saying "I'm sorry".

For more than 70 years we have always been trusted to play a unique part in the lives of our customers. If it's important to you, it's important to us.

Our commitment to excellence in every aspect of our business – from the beauty of a handcrafted floral arrangement to the delivery to your door – has only strengthened during our long and proud history in Australia. And we'll continue to do so, well into the future.

We don't just deliver flowers, but a feeling, a moment and an emotion. Because the act of giving and receiving flowers makes every moment brighter. Always.

#AlwaysInterflora

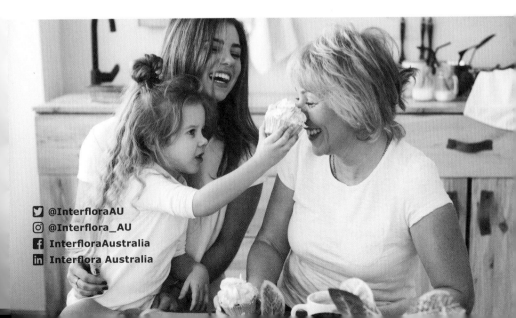

@InterfloraAU
@Interflora_AU
InterfloraAustralia
Interflora Australia

APRIL

S	M	T	W	T	F	S
	1	2	3	4	5	6
7	8	9	10	11	12	13
14	15	16	17	18	19	20
21	22	23	24	25	26	27
28	29	30				

MAY

S	M	T	W	T	F	S
			1	2	3	4
5	6	7	8	9	10	11
12	13	14	15	16	17	18
19	20	21	22	23	24	25
26	27	28	29	30	31	

JUNE

S	M	T	W	T	F	S
30						1
2	3	4	5	6	7	8
9	10	11	12	13	14	15
16	17	18	19	20	21	22
23	24	25	26	27	28	29

29 MONDAY

30 TUESDAY

1 WEDNESDAY

2 THURSDAY

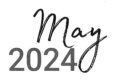

May
2024

3 FRIDAY

4 SATURDAY

5 SUNDAY ORTHODOX EASTER

	A P R I L					
S	M	T	W	T	F	S
	1	2	3	4	5	6
7	8	9	10	11	12	13
14	15	16	17	18	19	20
21	22	23	24	25	26	27
28	29	30				

	M A Y					
S	M	T	W	T	F	S
			1	2	3	4
5	6	7	8	9	10	11
12	13	14	15	16	17	18
19	20	21	22	23	24	25
26	27	28	29	30	31	

	J U N E					
S	M	T	W	T	F	S
30						1
2	3	4	5	6	7	8
9	10	11	12	13	14	15
16	17	18	19	20	21	22
23	24	25	26	27	28	29

6 MONDAY   LABOUR DAY (QLD), MAY DAY (NT)

7 TUESDAY

8 WEDNESDAY

9 THURSDAY

10 FRIDAY

11 SATURDAY

THE SIGNS OF POOR HEART HEALTH aren't always obvious, so it's important to have regular visits with your GP to monitor your blood pressure, blood glucose and cholesterol levels.

12 SUNDAY MOTHER'S DAY

		A P R I L				
S	M	T	W	T	F	S
	1	2	3	4	5	6
7	8	9	10	11	12	13
14	15	16	17	18	19	20
21	22	23	24	25	26	27
28	29	30				

		M A Y				
S	M	T	W	T	F	S
			1	2	3	4
5	6	7	8	9	10	11
12	13	14	15	16	17	18
19	20	21	22	23	24	25
26	27	28	29	30	31	

		J U N E				
S	M	T	W	T	F	S
30						1
2	3	4	5	6	7	8
9	10	11	12	13	14	15
16	17	18	19	20	21	22
23	24	25	26	27	28	29

13 MONDAY

14 TUESDAY

15 WEDNESDAY

16 THURSDAY

17 FRIDAY

18 SATURDAY

RESISTANCE TRAINING can help shift excess fat from around your middle for improved heart health. Try using hand weights or resistance bands on two non-consecutive days per week.

19 SUNDAY

APRIL						
S	M	T	W	T	F	S
	1	2	3	4	5	6
7	8	9	10	11	12	13
14	15	16	17	18	19	20
21	22	23	24	25	26	27
28	29	30				

MAY						
S	M	T	W	T	F	S
			1	2	3	4
5	6	7	8	9	10	11
12	13	14	15	16	17	18
19	20	21	22	23	24	25
26	27	28	29	30	31	

JUNE						
S	M	T	W	T	F	S
30						1
2	3	4	5	6	7	8
9	10	11	12	13	14	15
16	17	18	19	20	21	22
23	24	25	26	27	28	29

20 MONDAY

21 TUESDAY

22 WEDNESDAY

23 THURSDAY

24 FRIDAY

25 SATURDAY

ENDORPHINS (THE HAPPY HORMONES) are great for the heart. Trigger their release with exercise, stretching, deep breathing or by watching a romantic comedy movie.

26 SUNDAY NATIONAL SORRY DAY

		APRIL				
S	M	T	W	T	F	S
	1	2	3	4	5	6
7	8	9	10	11	12	13
14	15	16	17	18	19	20
21	22	23	24	25	26	27
28	29	30				

		MAY				
S	M	T	W	T	F	S
			1	2	3	4
5	6	7	8	9	10	11
12	13	14	15	16	17	18
19	20	21	22	23	24	25
26	27	28	29	30	31	

		JUNE				
S	M	T	W	T	F	S
30						1
2	3	4	5	6	7	8
9	10	11	12	13	14	15
16	17	18	19	20	21	22
23	24	25	26	27	28	29

27 MONDAY RECONCILIATION DAY (ACT)

28 TUESDAY

29 WEDNESDAY

30 THURSDAY

May–June 2024

31 FRIDAY

1 SATURDAY

2 SUNDAY

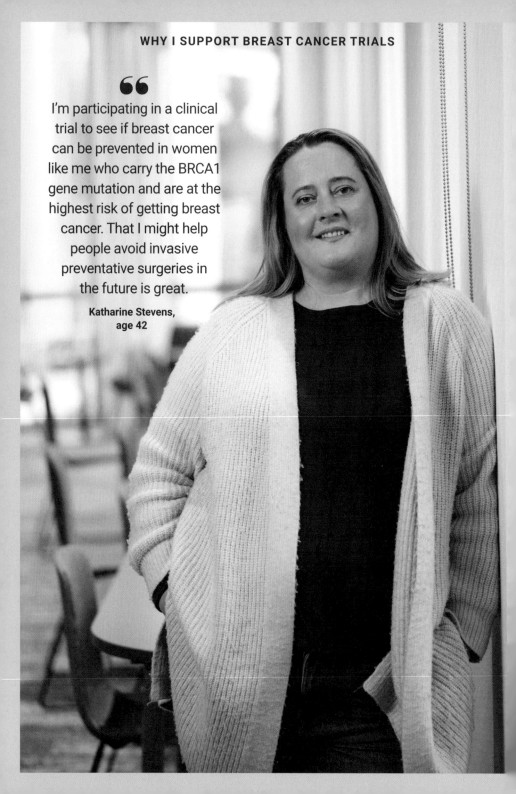

66

I'm participating in a clinical trial to see if breast cancer can be prevented in women like me who carry the BRCA1 gene mutation and are at the highest risk of getting breast cancer. That I might help people avoid invasive preventative surgeries in the future is great.

Katharine Stevens, age 42

let's talk about
YOUR FINANCES

It's never too late to take control of your financial health and future, by making smart spending decisions, working to reduce debt, setting up a sustainable budget and planning for a rainy day.

In today's tech-driven society, cyber fraud, scams and data leaks can affect us all. Recent data from the Australian Bureau of Statistics reveals two-thirds of Australians aged 15 and over were exposed to a scam in 2021-22, many of which were of a financial nature. Scams target people of all backgrounds, ages and income levels, with many scams extremely convincing. But the good news is there are a number of steps you can take to protect yourself from these threats.

SIMPLE WAYS TO AVOID SCAMS

- **Be alert.** Whenever you receive an unexpected phone call, email or text message, always consider the possibility that the sender may not be who they say they are. Do your research or check directly with the supposed source.
- **Never share personal details,** click on links or open attachments from unsolicited sources, or allow a stranger access to your computer or phone. No bank or institution will call, email or text asking for your bank details or credit card number.
- **If you're unsure** if a request is legitimate, tell a friend, family member or neighbour. They might be able to spot a telltale warning sign that you missed.
- **Choose passwords carefully.** They should be difficult for others to guess – a mix of upper and lowercase letters, numbers and symbols is always recommended. Avoid using the same password for every account and device, and try to change them every three months.
- **Utilise two-factor or multi-factor authentication** (for example, a password followed by a unique code) on your phone, computer, email, internet banking, social media and anywhere else it's offered. This provides stronger protection against unauthorised users.
- **Use social media security and privacy settings** so only your close friends and contacts can see what you share. And be careful what you post on these platforms – avoid sharing personal details like your address, date of birth, work history or other information that could be used to identify or manipulate you.

IF YOU SUSPECT YOU'VE BEEN ON THE RECEIVING END OF A SCAM or that your personal information has been illegally accessed, report it to the police or the relevant organisation or financial institution straightaway.

For more information, visit Scamwatch; scamwatch.gov.au

Healthy dinner ideas on a budget

With the cost of groceries on the rise, serving nutritious dinners on a budget may seem an impossible ask. To keep costs down, make a weekly meal plan using what's already in your fridge and pantry; buy fruit and vegetables in season; choose home brand products, canned vegetables and frozen fruit; and cook from scratch. Try these economic options.

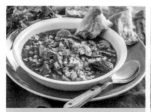

BEEF & BARLEY SOUP Slow-cook a cheap cut of meat like chuck steak or beef brisket in stock with barley and any vegetables on hand.

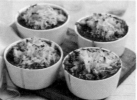

COTTAGE PIES Brown beef mince, onion, celery and carrot, add a can of tomatoes and simmer. Top with mashed potato or parsnip.

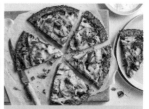

HOMEMADE PIZZA Making your own costs less than takeaway. Try homemade sauce, cooked chicken, red onion, capsicum and cheese.

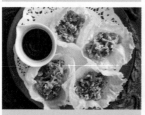

SAN CHOY BOW In a wok, fry pork mince, garlic, ginger and shallots. Add a splash of oyster sauce and low-salt soy. Serve in lettuce cups.

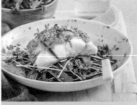

MISO FISH Combine miso paste, garlic, ginger and mirin to form a paste. Spread on top of firm white fish fillets and bake until just cooked.

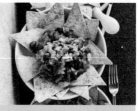

VEGETARIAN NACHOS Saute garlic, onion, capsicum, kidney beans, tomatoes and taco seasoning. Serve with homemade pita chips.

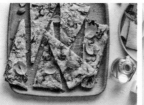

VEGIE FRITTATA Roast red onion, capsicum and pumpkin until soft. Add to a baking dish and top with whisked eggs and herbs and cook.

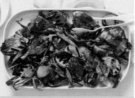

BALSAMIC CHICKEN Marinate chicken drumsticks with balsamic vinegar, garlic and herbs and bake until cooked. Serve with salad.

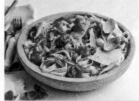

TUNA FETTUCCINE Make a sauce from tomatoes, onion, basil and chilli flakes, mix in a can of tuna and toss through wholemeal pasta.

Dealing with debt

If you currently owe money or are falling behind on repayments, you're not alone. Seventy-five per cent of Australian households are in debt, owing three or more times their annual disposable income. Credit cards are the most common source of debt, followed by home loans and student loans. Take these steps to tackle debt and seek help where needed.

STEP 1 Make a list of all your debts, including credit cards, mortgage repayments, student loans, personal loans, unpaid bills, fines, buy now pay later schemes, tax debts and so on. Include the full amount that's owed, the minimum monthly repayment (if any) and when payments are due. Add up the total amount and try not to be discouraged – you are on the way to taking back control of your money.

STEP 2 Work out how much (if anything) you can afford to pay each month to reduce these debts. Take a good look at what you've been spending money on and decide what you can cut back on or cancel altogether. Once you have a figure you can commit to, use it to pay the minimum amount on as many debts as you can, prioritising essentials like rent or the mortgage and those with higher interest rates, such as credit cards.

STEP 3 If you cannot manage any of your repayments, speak to your lenders or creditors as soon as possible and work together to negotiate a reasonable repayment arrangement that you can stick to. This will often eliminate the involvement of debt collectors.

STEP 4 If you can't afford to pay anything at all, seek advice from a financial counsellor or get confidential help by calling the National Debt Helpline on 1800 007 007 or the Mob Strong Debt Helpline for Aboriginal and Torres Strait Islander people on 1800 808 488.

> **REMEMBER, many banks and credit card companies have hardship teams who may be able to reduce, delay or waive repayments. The sooner you notify them of your situation, the more assistance they can give you.**

URGENT SUPPORT If you're struggling to make ends meet, there are plenty of services and organisations that can help you.

- Your local community centre, church, Salvation Army or St Vincent de Paul Society branch can provide assistance in the form of groceries, transport vouchers, housing, clothing or furniture, and help with bills, school costs and emotional support.
- Centrelink has various provisions available to those who need income support, are experiencing financial hardship or have been affected by a natural disaster. Call 132 850 or apply through the myGov app.
- Your state or territory housing department can assist with temporary and financially assisted accommodation for those in need.
- Seek emotional support from Lifeline (131 114) or your GP.

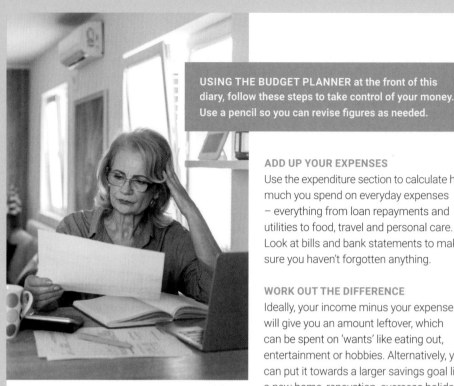

USING THE BUDGET PLANNER at the front of this diary, follow these steps to take control of your money. Use a pencil so you can revise figures as needed.

How to create a budget

Having a budget allows you to monitor your spending and work towards achieving those savings goals. By comparing your incoming funds with outgoing expenses you can clamp down on overspending and find extra money to put towards the things that matter to you. Here's how.

RECORD YOUR INCOME

Your income is essentially any money that comes into your account from wages, pensions, investments or government benefits. Use the columns provided to note down how much this equates to weekly, monthly and annually, or if you don't have a regular income, check last year's tax return to get an average figure. You may like to include your partner's income here if you have shared accounts.

ADD UP YOUR EXPENSES

Use the expenditure section to calculate how much you spend on everyday expenses – everything from loan repayments and utilities to food, travel and personal care. Look at bills and bank statements to make sure you haven't forgotten anything.

WORK OUT THE DIFFERENCE

Ideally, your income minus your expenses will give you an amount leftover, which can be spent on 'wants' like eating out, entertainment or hobbies. Alternatively, you can put it towards a larger savings goal like a new home, renovation, overseas holiday or topping up your superannuation. If you're spending more than you earn, go back to your expenses and consider ways you may be able to reduce this figure down.

ALLOW FOR A RAINY DAY

It's always good to have some money set aside for those unexpected expenses like home or mechanical repairs, medical bills or vet emergencies. You may like to transfer some of your leftover money into a separate high-interest savings account where you can still access it as needed. Set up a direct debit so it goes in automatically.

REVIEW YOUR BUDGET

Living expenses change and so might your money goals, so it's important to revisit your budget on a regular basis. This could be at the end of each month or at the end of each financial year.

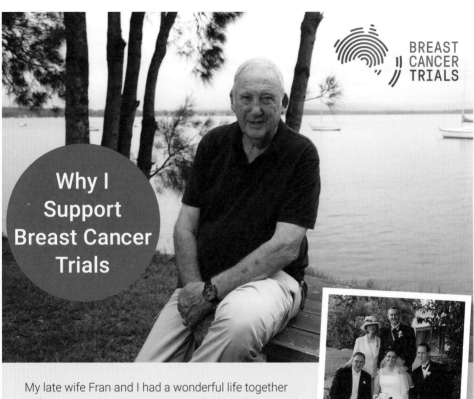

Why I Support Breast Cancer Trials

Paul and Fran on their son's wedding day

My late wife Fran and I had a wonderful life together with our sons, but it came to an end when she passed away from breast cancer at age 60.

When anyone goes through this or watches their cherished loved one go through it and see your family and its dreams for the future destroyed, you just can't say 'why us?' and do nothing about it.

I have chosen to leave a gift in my will to Breast Cancer Trials because I'm convinced that well-funded research will find solutions so that no more women of any age will suffer the indignities and pain of breast cancer, and the devastation it causes families like mine will stop.

No one fought harder than my late wife, and I'm not going to stop fighting because she never gave up and I'm not going to either.

FIND OUT THE POWERFUL LEGACY A GIFT TO BREAST CANCER TRIALS IN YOUR WILL CAN MAKE. GO TO BREASTCANCERTRIALS.ORG.AU, PHONE 1800 423 444 OR SCAN THIS QR CODE.

		MAY								JUNE							JULY			
S	M	T	W	T	F	S	S	M	T	W	T	F	S	S	M	T	W	T	F	S
			1	2	3	4	30						1		1	2	3	4	5	6
5	6	7	8	9	10	11	2	3	4	5	6	7	8	7	8	9	10	11	12	13
12	13	14	15	16	17	18	9	10	11	12	13	14	15	14	15	16	17	18	19	20
19	20	21	22	23	24	25	16	17	18	19	20	21	22	21	22	23	24	25	26	27
26	27	28	29	30	31		23	24	25	26	27	28	29	28	29	30	31			

3 MONDAY WESTERN AUSTRALIA DAY (WA)

4 TUESDAY

5 WEDNESDAY

6 THURSDAY

7 FRIDAY

8 SATURDAY

TAKE A MONEY MINUTE. Spend 60 seconds every day checking your bank balance and credit card transactions to stay on top of your financial health.

9 SUNDAY

MAY

S	M	T	W	T	F	S
				1	2	3	4
5	6	7	8	9	10	11
12	13	14	15	16	17	18
19	20	21	22	23	24	25
26	27	28	29	30	31	

JUNE

S	M	T	W	T	F	S
30						1
2	3	4	5	6	7	8
9	10	11	12	13	14	15
16	17	18	19	20	21	22
23	24	25	26	27	28	29

JULY

S	M	T	W	T	F	S
	1	2	3	4	5	6
7	8	9	10	11	12	13
14	15	16	17	18	19	20
21	22	23	24	25	26	27
28	29	30	31			

10 MONDAY KING'S BIRTHDAY (ACT, NSW, NT, SA, TAS, VIC)

11 TUESDAY

12 WEDNESDAY

13 THURSDAY

14 FRIDAY

15 SATURDAY

LIMIT TAKEAWAY TO REAP INSTANT SAVINGS. Make your coffee at home, have last night's dinner leftovers for lunch and make your own pizza, burgers or curries to satisfy fast food cravings.

16 SUNDAY

			MAY								JUNE								JULY			
S	M	T	W	T	F	S		S	M	T	W	T	F	S		S	M	T	W	T	F	S
				1	2	3	4	30						1			1	2	3	4	5	6
5	6	7	8	9	10	11		2	3	4	5	6	7	8		7	8	9	10	11	12	13
12	13	14	15	16	17	18		9	10	11	12	13	14	15		14	15	16	17	18	19	20
19	20	21	22	23	24	25		16	17	18	19	20	21	22		21	22	23	24	25	26	27
26	27	28	29	30	31			23	24	25	26	27	28	29		28	29	30	31			

17 MONDAY EID AL-ADHA (ISLAMIC HOLIDAY)

18 TUESDAY

19 WEDNESDAY

20 THURSDAY

21 FRIDAY

22 SATURDAY

23 SUNDAY

MAY						
S	M	T	W	T	F	S
				1	2	3	4
5	6	7	8	9	10	11
12	13	14	15	16	17	18
19	20	21	22	23	24	25
26	27	28	29	30	31	

JUNE						
S	M	T	W	T	F	S
30						1
2	3	4	5	6	7	8
9	10	11	12	13	14	15
16	17	18	19	20	21	22
23	24	25	26	27	28	29

JULY						
S	M	T	W	T	F	S
	1	2	3	4	5	6
7	8	9	10	11	12	13
14	15	16	17	18	19	20
21	22	23	24	25	26	27
28	29	30	31			

24 MONDAY

25 TUESDAY

26 WEDNESDAY

27 THURSDAY

June
2024

28 FRIDAY

29 SATURDAY

30 SUNDAY

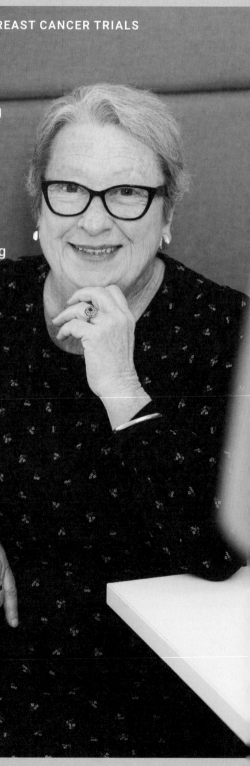

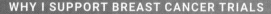

66

When I was first diagnosed 15 years ago, I remember feeling thankful for the treatments available. I soon realised the treatments were enabled by the many patients who had participated in previous clinical trials. My breast cancer has returned and I'm now participating in a trial myself. I feel blessed that I'm responding well.

Madelaine Atkins,
first diagnosed at age 50

let's talk about
AGEING

Our physical, dietary and mental health needs all shift significantly as we get older and face new medical challenges and a change in life stage. Prepare for these changes to enjoy life to its fullest.

Our risk of sustaining a fracture increases with age, and becomes more of a concern for those with chronic conditions like arthritis and osteoporosis. Try these tips to reduce your falls risk.

STRATEGY #1 Exercise safely
Regular exercise improves muscle tone, strength and balance, but should always be undertaken with your doctor's advice. They may suggest yoga, Pilates or Tai Chi for balance and flexibility, or using weights or resistance bands to build strength.

STRATEGY #2 Fall-proof your home
Install handrails on stairs and grab rails in bathrooms, use non-slip mats, keep walkways clear of clutter, clean up spills immediately and replace broken or uneven floor tiles. Also make sure your home is well lit so you can see where you're going.

STRATEGY #3 Look after your feet
Sore, tired feet can affect the way we walk, so see a podiatrist for advice. Shoes with a broad heel, non-slip sole and good support are ideal for balance. Avoid loose-fitting slippers, thongs or scuffs, and wear socks with shoes to reduce your falls risk.

STRATEGY #4 Test hearing and eyesight
Hearing and sight loss can both increase the risk of falls. Have your eyes tested every year by an optometrist and wear glasses as directed. Likewise, have your hearing checked annually after the age of 65, and if needed, get fitted for a hearing aid.

STRATEGY #5 Manage medications
It's important to take medications as prescribed and always inform your GP of any new drugs you are taking or if a medicine is making you feel drowsy or light-headed.

STRATEGY #6 Avoid or limit alcohol
Age makes us more vulnerable to the effects of alcohol, which can lead to poor spatial awareness, coordination problems and lack of balance. Reduce your intake to stay steady on your feet.

STRATEGY #7 Use support when needed
If you feel unstable on your feet, consider using a cane or walker for assistance. Your doctor, physiotherapist or occupational therapist can help you decide which support device is best for your needs and teach you how to use it properly. Always make sure it's the right size and height for you.

For more information, visit Healthy Bones Australia; healthybonesaustralia.org.au

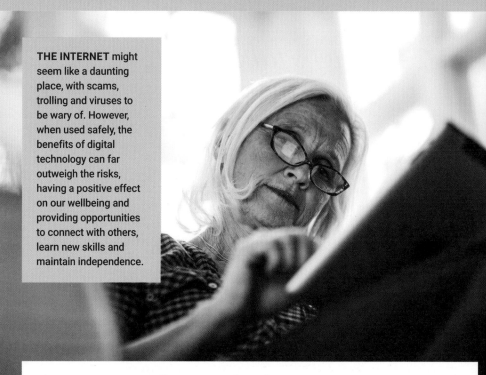

THE INTERNET might seem like a daunting place, with scams, trolling and viruses to be wary of. However, when used safely, the benefits of digital technology can far outweigh the risks, having a positive effect on our wellbeing and providing opportunities to connect with others, learn new skills and maintain independence.

5 reasons to embrace technology

1 Social connection
We can combat loneliness and isolation by using video calling apps like FaceTime and Zoom to chat with loved ones, sharing photos through Instagram or keeping abreast of family happenings through WhatsApp.

2 Access to information
Being online gives us instant access to news and current events, not to mention the ability to stream music, movies and TV shows through a smartphone, iPad or TV. There are also millions of recipes, online courses and podcasts available at your fingertips.

3 Convenience
Many everyday tasks can be done online, from ordering groceries to paying bills and making restaurant bookings. This can be helpful for those who live in remote locations, have mobility issues or want to avoid crowds. Smart home technology also makes tasks, such as vacuuming, turning on lights or answering the doorbell, that much easier.

4 Better brain health
Challenging your mind with online games like Wordle, Solitaire or Sudoku can help lower the chances of neurological decline and improve memory and spatial recognition. Digital jigsaws are also great for mindfulness.

5 Access to health services
Many doctors and specialists provide a telehealth option over the computer or phone for patients who cannot manage face-to-face appointments. You can also use apps to track medications, check symptoms via the Healthdirect symptom checker and utilise e-scripts at your local pharmacy.

The perks of retirement

The prospect of retiring can be both exciting and daunting – you may worry you'll be bored, lonely or lose your sense of purpose. But retirement can in fact provide new opportunities and greater flexibility. Here are just some of the things to look forward to.

TRAVEL One of the biggest perks of retirement is having the time to travel at your own pace. Whether you book an overseas cruise, hit the road in a motorhome or explore your local area, the world is your oyster.

BETTER HEALTH When you were working, you may not have had the time or energy to exercise or cook nutritious meals, but now you do. See your GP for check-ups, book in for a massage or try a new fitness class.

REVIVED RELATIONSHIPS Now's the time to reconnect with your partner and friends, particularly if your children have also left the nest. Go for walks, eat out or pursue common interests, without work pressures interfering.

FAMILY TIME With more time on your hands, relish the opportunity to spend quality time with your children or grandchildren. Attend sports games and performances, offer to babysit or organise a family holiday.

NEW SKILLS & INTERESTS You're never too old to learn something new. Master a new language, study your family tree, take a dance class or learn to play an instrument.

GREATER SOCIAL OPPORTUNITIES There are numerous groups, clubs or organisations that you can join (often for free) to meet new people and participate in social outings and activities. Check with your local council or library for options near you.

GIVING BACK Now's the time to be more active in your local community. Why not volunteer at your local sporting club, library, hospital or animal shelter, host a fundraising event or become a mentor to local youth?

GOVERNMENT BENEFITS Once you turn 60, you may be eligible for government benefits to help reduce the cost of living. These might include discounts on public transport, meals or healthcare, plus access to energy rebates, aged care assistance and rental assistance.

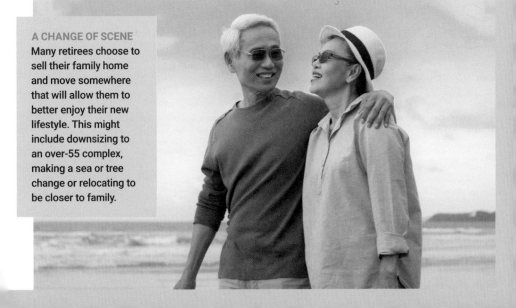

A CHANGE OF SCENE
Many retirees choose to sell their family home and move somewhere that will allow them to better enjoy their new lifestyle. This might include downsizing to an over-55 complex, making a sea or tree change or relocating to be closer to family.

Healthy eating after 50

As we get older, the way and the amount we eat can change dramatically. Inactivity, decreasing appetite, lifestyle changes, chronic health conditions and food aversions can all have an impact on our dietary choices. But despite all this, our nutritional requirements stay the same or, in some cases, increase. Keep the following in mind to meet all your nutritional needs.

FOLLOW THE DIETARY GUIDELINES
For women over 50, the daily recommendations are as follows:

- 5 serves of vegetables
- 2 serves of fruit
- 4 serves of grains and cereals (down from 6 serves previously)
- 2 serves of lean meat, poultry, fish, eggs, tofu, nuts, seeds or legumes
- 4 serves of dairy or dairy alternatives (up from 2.5 serves previously)

Eat a range of foods across the five food groups to get a variety of vitamins and minerals. Change one thing at a time – the fruit on your muesli, the bread in your sandwich or a new vegetable with your fish.

Limit salty and sugary food and drink. Pies, pastries, fried and battered foods, chips, biscuits, ice cream and chocolate should only be eaten very occasionally as they're usually high in saturated fat, and in some cases, trans fats. Soft drink, cordial and fruit juice are also high in sugar.

Make use of meal-delivery services. If you find it hard to get to the shops or have lost interest in cooking, having nutritionally balanced meals delivered to your door by the likes of Meals on Wheels or Lite n' Easy can ensure you're still eating well.

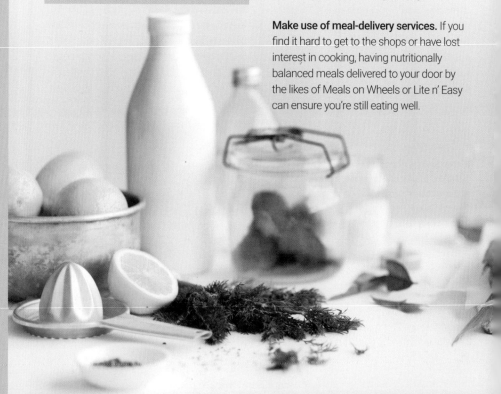

Keep it simple. While variety is important, food aversions and malnutrition may be an issue for some. Choose meals that are simple to prepare, and feel free to resort to nourishing comfort foods. Try baked beans or sardines on toast, thick and hearty canned soup (look for a low sodium content) or a grazing plate of cheese, crackers and fruit.

Drink more water. Dehydration can become more of an issue when we get older, as we may not feel thirsty as often. Aim to drink at least six cups of water and other fluids like tea, milk and soda water each day, and more in warmer weather or if you're exercising.

Include plenty of fibre. This will also help prevent constipation. Wholegrain cereals, wholemeal bread, fruit, vegetables, beans and legumes are all excellent forms of fibre.

Look after your teeth. If nuts, grains and hard fruits and vegetables are difficult to chew, try nut pastes and butters, baked beans and cooked and canned fruit and vegetables.

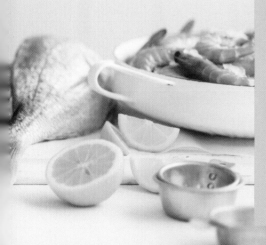

UTIs in the elderly

A urinary tract infection (UTI) is an infection that can affect the urethra, ureters, bladder and kidneys. UTIs are more prevalent in women and are also one of the most common infections in older adults, with more than 10 per cent of women aged 65 and over contracting one in the last 12 months. The symptoms in seniors can also be more severe.

WHY ARE THE ELDERLY MORE AT RISK?

As we age, the tissues of our urethra become thinner and drier, particularly after menopause. Constipation, incontinence and chronic conditions (such as diabetes) can also make us more susceptible to UTIs.

WHAT ARE THE COMPLICATIONS?

The usual symptoms of a UTI include: a burning sensation when passing urine; wanting to urinate more often; cloudy, bloody or smelly urine; pain above the pubic bone; fatigue, fever and chills. However, older adults are more likely to experience extreme changes in behaviour, such as confusion and irritation, or may be more prone to falls. If left untreated, the infection can spread to the kidneys and cause life-threatening sepsis, so always see a doctor if you have any symptoms, to avoid these serious complications.

HOW CAN UTIs BE PREVENTED?

Lower your risk by drinking lots of fluids, particularly water, to wash unwanted bacteria from the bladder and urinary tract. Eat a healthy balanced diet with plenty of fibre to prevent constipation. Always wipe front to back when using the toilet, take your time and try to empty your bladder completely.

For more information, visit the Continence Foundation of Australia; continence.org.au

	J U N E					
S	M	T	W	T	F	S
30						1
2	3	4	5	6	7	8
9	10	11	12	13	14	15
16	17	18	19	20	21	22
23	24	25	26	27	28	29

	J U L Y					
S	M	T	W	T	F	S
	1	2	3	4	5	6
7	8	9	10	11	12	13
14	15	16	17	18	19	20
21	22	23	24	25	26	27
28	29	30	31			

	A U G U S T					
S	M	T	W	T	F	S
				1	2	3
4	5	6	7	8	9	10
11	12	13	14	15	16	17
18	19	20	21	22	23	24
25	26	27	28	29	30	31

1 MONDAY

2 TUESDAY

3 WEDNESDAY

4 THURSDAY

5 FRIDAY

6 SATURDAY

NEED TO BRUSH UP ON YOUR DIGITAL SKILLS? Visit beconnected. esafety.gov.au to access free online courses, resources and important cyber safety tips.

7 SUNDAY NAIDOC WEEK BEGINS

			JUNE								JULY								AUGUST			
S	M	T	W	T	F	S		S	M	T	W	T	F	S		S	M	T	W	T	F	S
30						1			1	2	3	4	5	6						1	2	3
2	3	4	5	6	7	8		7	8	9	10	11	12	13		4	5	6	7	8	9	10
9	10	11	12	13	14	15		14	15	16	17	18	19	20		11	12	13	14	15	16	17
16	17	18	19	20	21	22		21	22	23	24	25	26	27		18	19	20	21	22	23	24
23	24	25	26	27	28	29		28	29	30	31					25	26	27	28	29	30	31

8 MONDAY   MUHARRAM/ISLAMIC NEW YEAR

9 TUESDAY

10 WEDNESDAY

11 THURSDAY

12 FRIDAY

13 SATURDAY

VITAMIN D HELPS KEEP MUSCLES STRONG and assists with calcium absorption. Ask your GP for a blood test to check your levels; supplements may be needed.

14 SUNDAY BASTILLE DAY (FRANCE)

		JUNE				
S	M	T	W	T	F	S
30						1
2	3	4	5	6	7	8
9	10	11	12	13	14	15
16	17	18	19	20	21	22
23	24	25	26	27	28	29

		JULY				
S	M	T	W	T	F	S
	1	2	3	4	5	6
7	8	9	10	11	12	13
14	15	16	17	18	19	20
21	22	23	24	25	26	27
28	29	30	31			

		AUGUST				
S	M	T	W	T	F	S
				1	2	3
4	5	6	7	8	9	10
11	12	13	14	15	16	17
18	19	20	21	22	23	24
25	26	27	28	29	30	31

15 MONDAY

16 TUESDAY

17 WEDNESDAY

18 THURSDAY

19 FRIDAY

20 SATURDAY

FISH IS YOUR FRIEND. Regularly consuming fish may reduce your risk of heart disease, stroke, dementia and some types of vision loss. Aim to eat fish twice a week.

21 SUNDAY

		J U N E				
S	M	T	W	T	F	S
30						1
2	3	4	5	6	7	8
9	10	11	12	13	14	15
16	17	18	19	20	21	22
23	24	25	26	27	28	29

		J U L Y				
S	M	T	W	T	F	S
	1	2	3	4	5	6
7	8	9	10	11	12	13
14	15	16	17	18	19	20
21	22	23	24	25	26	27
28	29	30	31			

		A U G U S T				
S	M	T	W	T	F	S
				1	2	3
4	5	6	7	8	9	10
11	12	13	14	15	16	17
18	19	20	21	22	23	24
25	26	27	28	29	30	31

22 MONDAY

23 TUESDAY

24 WEDNESDAY

25 THURSDAY

26 FRIDAY

27 SATURDAY

> **SET UP A GROUP CHAT** with your extended family in Messenger or WhatsApp where you can all share your day-to-day experiences and photos.

28 SUNDAY

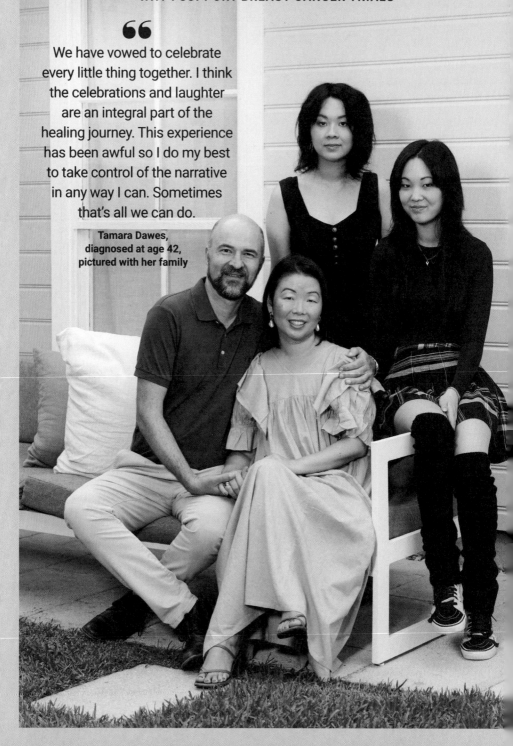

66

We have vowed to celebrate every little thing together. I think the celebrations and laughter are an integral part of the healing journey. This experience has been awful so I do my best to take control of the narrative in any way I can. Sometimes that's all we can do.

**Tamara Dawes,
diagnosed at age 42,
pictured with her family**

let's talk about
FAMILY

Family life can be equally rewarding and challenging, and our busy lives often make it difficult to stay on top of our loved ones' varying needs. Read on for helpful tips and techniques for all age groups.

Good communication is crucial for building strong family relationships, allowing each member to feel seen, heard, understood and supported. Here's how to improve your communication style.

Don't rush important conversations Set aside an adequate amount of time to talk without distractions. For the kids, this might be at mealtimes, in the car or before bedtime. Deeper conversations with your partner could happen at the end of the day or while going for a walk. And checking in with your parents or older children might be done on the phone or over coffee.

Ask open-ended questions Encourage family members to open up by avoiding questions that will illicit yes or no responses. For example, rather than asking, "Did you have a good day at school?", try "How was your day?" or "What was the most interesting thing that happened today?"

Listen first, then answer We're all guilty of tuning out when others speak, or biding time until we can have our say. Instead, listen carefully to what is being said then take a moment to process before responding. Establish a natural flow of back and forth, so no one is dominating the conversation and both parties feel valued.

Pay attention to your wording If you're saying "I" a lot, the conversation may be a little one-sided, and you should turn it back to your loved one to give them a chance to speak. Saying "You" a lot could come across as accusatory. Rather than "You really upset me when..." try "I feel upset when...".

Offer validation Not all conversations need advice or a fix. Sometimes a simple "That sounds so frustrating" or "I know exactly what you mean" is the perfect response.

Pick up on non-verbal cues Communication isn't just about the words that are said, but how they're said. Listen to the person's tone of voice and watch their facial expressions and body language to gauge what they may be feeling but aren't ready or able to say, and tailor your response accordingly.

Tell them you love them Never assume your loved ones know how much you value them – tell them, and tell them often. "Thank you for being such a good listener", "I love our time together" or "I'm so proud to be your mum/wife/sister/daughter" are just some examples of how you can express your love.

For more information, visit Relationships Australia; relationships.org.au

First aid at home

Accidents happen, even within the perceived safety of home. Be prepared by keeping a well-stocked first aid kit in a designated spot at home and in the car, and consider taking a basic first-aid course and learning CPR through the likes of St John Ambulance Australia and CPR Kids. For everyday minor injuries, this guide may help.

BURNS

For mild or superficial burns, hold under cold running water for 20 minutes and remove any clothing or jewellery from burnt area. Cover burn with a light, loose, non-stick dressing. Seek medical attention if burn appears infected. If the burn is severe or involves the airway, call Triple Zero (000).

MINOR CUTS & ABRASIONS

Wash the area with clean water or saline and gently pat dry. Cover with a dressing or adhesive plaster, and change daily. Seek medical attention if the area becomes hot to the touch, red or swollen. If bleeding is severe, you can see bone or deep tissue, there's an object imbedded in the wound or it was caused by an animal, apply pressure and go to hospital or call Triple Zero (000).

CONCUSSION

After a blow to the head, follow the DRSABCD action plan (Danger, Response, Send, Airway, Breathing, CPR, Defibrillation). If the patient is unconscious and breathing, place them into the recovery position and call Triple Zero (000) for an ambulance. If the patient is conscious, monitor closely and seek medical attention for the following: headache or neck pain; nausea/vomiting; drowsiness/fatigue; confusion, disorientation or memory loss; blurred vision or slurred speech; tingling in the arms or legs; seizures or loss of consciousness.

CHOKING

Call Triple Zero (000) for an ambulance and follow the operator's advice while you wait, which may include performing back blows or chest thrusts, as well as CPR.

NOSEBLEEDS

Ask the patient to sit with their head slightly forward (not back). Pinch nostril, applying pressure below the bridge of the nose for 10 minutes. Check if bleeding has stopped, otherwise repeat for another 10 minutes. Seek medical attention if bleeding persists or if patient is on blood-thinning medication.

SPRAINS & STRAINS

Follow the RICE protocol:
* Rest – rest the patient and the injured area.
* Ice – apply an ice pack or cold pack for 15 minutes every 2 hours for 24 hours, then 15 minutes every 4 hours for 24 hours.
* Compression – apply a compression bandage firmly to reduce swelling.
* Elevation – elevate the affected area.
Seek medical attention if pain persists.

SPIDER BITES

For a big black spider bite (funnel-web, mouse spider or large, black spiders), call Triple Zero (000), apply a pressure immobilisation bandage and keep the patient completely still while you wait for an ambulance. For all other spiders, wash the bite and apply a cold compress. If patient has difficulty breathing or swelling of the lips, face or mouth, seek urgent medical attention.

TICKS

Use an ether-containing aerosol, such as Wart-Off Freeze Spray, and allow tick to drop off naturally (avoid using tweezers, which may squeeze toxins into the bloodstream). Wash area; apply antiseptic and a plaster. See a doctor if there is a rash, swelling, infection or patient feels faint, sleepy, feverish or has difficulty breathing or swallowing.

For more first-aid advice, visit St John Ambulance Australia; stjohn.org.au

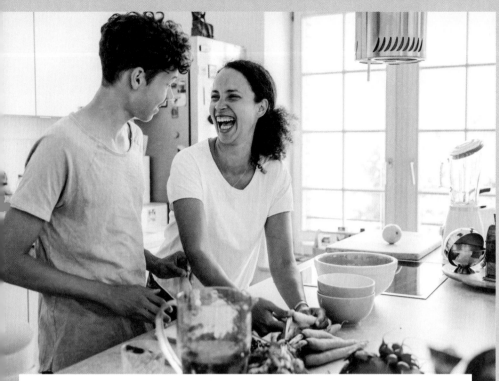

Simple hacks for stress-free family dinners

With busy schedules, budget constraints, varying nutritional needs and differing taste buds, feeding a family can be stressful. Try these strategies to make mealtimes work for you.

KEEP IT SIMPLE

A nutritious and delicious meal doesn't have to be expensive, complicated or Instagram-worthy. Choose simple recipes that use just a few ingredients.

NO FOOD IS OFF LIMITS

Foster a healthy relationship with food by avoiding labels like 'bad' or 'naughty'. All foods can be enjoyed in moderation: some (fruit and veg) every day and others (cake and chocolate) on occasion.

SHARE THE LOAD

Make meals a collaborative process. Young kids can wash vegies or set the table, while older kids can be in charge of cooking one meal each week or cleaning up. Ask everyone to nominate meal ideas each week to eliminate complaints.

REDUCE STRESS

If you have fussy eaters, avoid the daily battle by serving meals deconstructed, so each family member can pick and choose what they like. Tacos, wraps, stir-fries and pasta dishes all work well for this.

EMBRACE THE MICROWAVE

Older kids with evening commitments may not always be able to eat at the same time as you. Make one meal that can be reheated as needed. Casseroles, curries, soups, pasta bakes, lasagne or enchiladas are ideal.

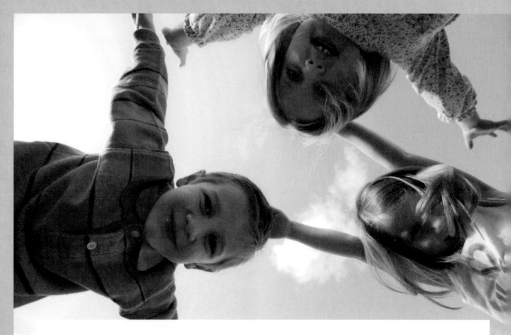

Embracing neurodiversity

Neurodiversity is a term used to describe the different ways in which our brains work. While a neurotypical individual will act or behave in a way that is typical for their age, a neurodivergent brain will veer outside of these parameters. Around one in five to six children have these natural variations in their brain ability, which can present as conditions like autism spectrum disorder (ASD), attention deficit hyperactivity disorder (ADHD), Tourette syndrome and obsessive compulsive disorder (OCD). A neurodivergent child's brain does not need to be 'fixed' or treated, but rather their difference should be celebrated and supported. Whether you have a neurodivergent child or want to teach your children to be inclusive, try these ideas:

- Learn more about neurodiversity and neurodivergence by reading online articles, joining Facebook groups or talking to neurodiverse adults. Be aware of the language you use, and don't be afraid to ask if you're not sure.
- Find meaningful ways to include neurodivergent children in social activities. For example, if you're inviting an autistic child for a play date, ask the parents how you can accommodate their child's needs.
- Avoid assumptions and 'labels'. There could be many reasons why a child is eating only packaged snacks at school or wearing headphones at the supermarket.
- Use books to learn and talk about neurodiversity. For young children, try *Some Brains* by Nelly Thomas or *The Brain Forest* by Sandhya Menon. For older children, try *The Autism and Neurodiversity Self Advocacy Handbook* by Barb Cook and Yenn Purkis.

Talk to your child about difference. Try putting it into terms they'll understand: "Some people's brains work differently to other people's. This means they learn and make friends differently."

For more information, visit Raising Children Network; raisingchildren.net.au

Technology tips for kids

From computers, televisions and phones, to apps, podcasts and social media, technology has become an integral part of our lives. This is particularly true for our children, who use technology to learn, play, communicate and socialise. As parents, it can be hard to know where to draw the line, however, we can create a framework for our family that balances technology use with other beneficial activities. Here's how.

1 SET CLEAR BOUNDARIES Work together to create a set of rules around technology in your house, including where, when and how it can be used.

2 BUILD IN REGULAR SCREEN BREAKS It's important for children to only use screens in short bursts and take regular breaks to eat, drink, stretch and move around. Set a timer or teach them to stop every time they reach a new level on a game or finish an episode of a TV show.

3 BALANCE IT OUT WITH MOVEMENT As well as screen breaks, children also need at least one hour of moderate to vigorous physical activity each day. This might be playing sport, walking or riding to school or taking part in organised activities like dancing, swimming or Nippers.

4 AVOID SCREENS BEFORE BED Primary school-aged children need nine to 11 hours of sleep each night, while teenagers should have eight to 10 hours, and using technology too close to bedtime can inhibit this. Ban phones and devices from bedrooms and have a switch-off time of at least one hour before bed.

5 ENCOURAGE SCREEN-FREE INTERESTS Extracurricular activities or hobbies provide kids with a chance to learn new skills and meet new people. Look into language classes, music, debating, photography, craft or groups like Scouts and Guides.

6 PRIORITISE FRIENDSHIPS Social media should never take the place of face-to-face interactions. Support your child's friendships by encouraging them to invite friends over and driving them to public meet-ups at the park, shops or movies.

7 BE A GOOD ROLE MODEL Studies have found a strong relationship between parent screen use and that of their children. To reduce how much time your children spend using technology, you should also apply the same rules to your own technology use.

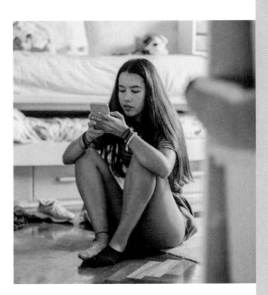

J U L Y						
S	M	T	W	T	F	S
	1	2	3	4	5	6
7	8	9	10	11	12	13
14	15	16	17	18	19	20
21	22	23	24	25	26	27
28	29	30	31			

A U G U S T						
S	M	T	W	T	F	S
					1	2	3
4	5	6	7	8	9	10
11	12	13	14	15	16	17
18	19	20	21	22	23	24
25	26	27	28	29	30	31

S E P T E M B E R						
S	M	T	W	T	F	S
1	2	3	4	5	6	7
8	9	10	11	12	13	14
15	16	17	18	19	20	21
22	23	24	25	26	27	28
29	30					

29 MONDAY

30 TUESDAY

31 WEDNESDAY

1 THURSDAY

August
2024

2 FRIDAY

3 SATURDAY

4 SUNDAY

		J U L Y				
S	M	T	W	T	F	S
	1	2	3	4	5	6
7	8	9	10	11	12	13
14	15	16	17	18	19	20
21	22	23	24	25	26	27
28	29	30	31			

		A U G U S T				
S	M	T	W	T	F	S
				1	2	3
4	5	6	7	8	9	10
11	12	13	14	15	16	17
18	19	20	21	22	23	24
25	26	27	28	29	30	31

	S E P T E M B E R					
S	M	T	W	T	F	S
1	2	3	4	5	6	7
8	9	10	11	12	13	14
15	16	17	18	19	20	21
22	23	24	25	26	27	28
29	30					

5 MONDAY   BANK HOLIDAY (NSW), PICNIC DAY (NT)

6 TUESDAY

7 WEDNESDAY

8 THURSDAY

August
2024

9 FRIDAY

10 SATURDAY

TEACH KIDS TO BE KIND ONLINE. Remind them not to say or do anything online that could hurt or humiliate others, and not to forward material that may embarrass or endanger someone else.

11 SUNDAY

JULY
S	M	T	W	T	F	S
	1	2	3	4	5	6
7	8	9	10	11	12	13
14	15	16	17	18	19	20
21	22	23	24	25	26	27
28	29	30	31			

AUGUST
S	M	T	W	T	F	S
				1	2	3
4	5	6	7	8	9	10
11	12	13	14	15	16	17
18	19	20	21	22	23	24
25	26	27	28	29	30	31

SEPTEMBER
S	M	T	W	T	F	S
1	2	3	4	5	6	7
8	9	10	11	12	13	14
15	16	17	18	19	20	21
22	23	24	25	26	27	28
29	30					

12 MONDAY

13 TUESDAY

14 WEDNESDAY

15 THURSDAY

August
2024

16 FRIDAY

17 SATURDAY

WRITTEN COMMUNICATION can be extremely powerful. Write your partner, child or parent a card or letter, which can be read over and over, to let them know just how much they mean to you.

18 SUNDAY

JULY

S	M	T	W	T	F	S
	1	2	3	4	5	6
7	8	9	10	11	12	13
14	15	16	17	18	19	20
21	22	23	24	25	26	27
28	29	30	31			

AUGUST

S	M	T	W	T	F	S
				1	2	3
4	5	6	7	8	9	10
11	12	13	14	15	16	17
18	19	20	21	22	23	24
25	26	27	28	29	30	31

SEPTEMBER

S	M	T	W	T	F	S
1	2	3	4	5	6	7
8	9	10	11	12	13	14
15	16	17	18	19	20	21
22	23	24	25	26	27	28
29	30					

19 MONDAY

20 TUESDAY

21 WEDNESDAY

22 THURSDAY

23 FRIDAY

24 SATURDAY

IN CASE OF EMERGENCY, staple a list of your child's medical conditions, allergies, and medications to their immunisation record. Keep copies in your purse and on the fridge, and take a photo of it to keep in your phone.

25 SUNDAY

JULY						
S	M	T	W	T	F	S
	1	2	3	4	5	6
7	8	9	10	11	12	13
14	15	16	17	18	19	20
21	22	23	24	25	26	27
28	29	30	31			

AUGUST						
S	M	T	W	T	F	S
					1	2	3
4	5	6	7	8	9	10
11	12	13	14	15	16	17
18	19	20	21	22	23	24
25	26	27	28	29	30	31

SEPTEMBER						
S	M	T	W	T	F	S
1	2	3	4	5	6	7
8	9	10	11	12	13	14
15	16	17	18	19	20	21
22	23	24	25	26	27	28
29	30					

26 MONDAY

27 TUESDAY

28 WEDNESDAY

29 THURSDAY

August–September
2024

30 FRIDAY

31 SATURDAY

IF YOU'RE PLANNING A PREGNANCY, make sure your immunisations against measles, mumps, rubella, chickenpox and whooping cough are up to date.

1 SUNDAY FATHER'S DAY

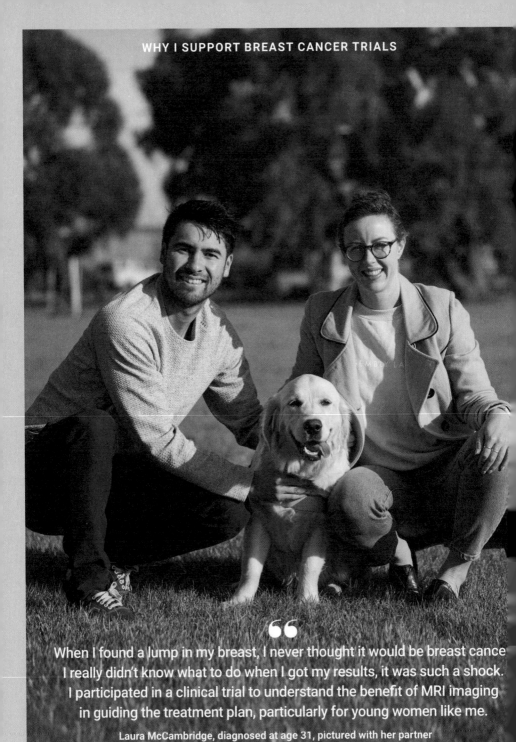

"

When I found a lump in my breast, I never thought it would be breast cancer
I really didn't know what to do when I got my results, it was such a shock.
I participated in a clinical trial to understand the benefit of MRI imaging
in guiding the treatment plan, particularly for young women like me.

Laura McCambridge, diagnosed at age 31, pictured with her partner

let's talk about
WELLBEING

Forty-four per cent of Australians aged 16-85 will experience a mental disorder like anxiety or depression at least once during their lives. Learn how to navigate life's hurdles and make your wellbeing top priority.

Having someone to share life's ups and downs with is extremely important for our mental health. Romantic partners, friends, neighbours, colleagues, carers and even pets can all play the role of companion and reduce unwanted feelings of social isolation, loneliness and despair. This applies to our elderly citizens most of all, who may find it difficult to keep up connections and maintain relationships due to mobility issues and living alone or away from family and friends. Try these suggestions to find that special someone and keep loneliness at bay.

Deepen casual connections
The neighbour you wave to across the road, the school mum who always smiles at the front gate, the regulars at your local cafe – these existing connections have great friendship potential. Take things further by inviting a casual acquaintance for a walk, a coffee or a chat, and you could end up with a lifelong friend.

Do what you love
The best way to meet someone with similar interests to you is to get out and do the things that bring you joy. Play a sport, start a book club, join a choir or take an art class. The workplace can also provide that same opportunity if you love what you do. Working alongside a group of colleagues with a shared passion or goals creates an incredibly strong bond that will often evolve into friendship.

Become a volunteer
Whether you're helping out at your child's or grandchild's school, volunteering at a hospital, mentoring young people or giving your time to a charity, you'll meet plenty of interesting people, some who could become firm friends. Plus, you'll get the added mental health benefits of greater purpose, self-esteem, happiness and satisfaction with life.

Get a pet
Animal companionship has been found to have numerous benefits for our mental wellbeing, social interactions and physical health. Pets provide a constant, calming presence, keeping us company if we're sick or sad and offering unconditional love, loyalty and affection. They make us feel needed and give us a sense of purpose each day. Plus, owning a dog provides opportunities for regular exercise and social interactions with fellow dog owners. Consider adopting from a local shelter.

What is addiction?

One of the most misunderstood chronic health conditions, addiction, occurs when someone is unable to stop doing or consuming something even though it is negatively affecting their physical and psychological wellbeing. Addiction does not discriminate, and can affect young and older people from all communities. In Australia, one in five people will experience problems with alcohol, drug use or gambling during their lifetime, and approximately 10 per cent of adult Australians are daily smokers. Breaking the habit can sometimes be harder to deal with than the addiction itself, so the cycle continues. In some cases, addiction may lead to relationship problems, financial difficulties, social withdrawal and job loss.

Why do people become addicted?

There are a number of psychological and environmental factors that can lead to addiction. In many cases, the substance (such as illicit drugs, alcohol, nicotine, solvents or prescription drugs) or activity (such as gambling, shopping or gaming) can make some people feel relaxed, happy, pain-free or confident. Over time, though, the pursuit of this 'feel good' factor can dominate a person's life. The substance or activity can also be used as a coping mechanism for difficult issues, such as poverty, stress, grief, unemployment or workplace pressure.

ARE PAINKILLERS ADDICTIVE?

Some prescription medicines contain active ingredients known as opioids. For example, codeine, fentanyl, morphine, methadone or oxycodone. Doctors can prescribe these as a necessary form of pain relief. However, there is a risk of becoming dependent on opioids, particularly when they're taken at a higher dose than what is prescribed. If a person has developed a dependence on opioids and stops using them suddenly, they are likely to experience withdrawal symptoms, such as cravings, anxiety, nausea, muscle aches and sleep disruptions. Speak to your doctor, who can provide information on how to reduce your risk of harm and dependence.

WHERE TO GET HELP

There is plenty of support available for people affected by addiction, but it's important to know that quitting can be a gradual process and can take several attempts. You might like to start by talking to your doctor, seeking support from family and friends or using one of many free and confidential support services, including:

Lifeline Australia 131 114; lifeline.org.au **The Alcohol and Drug Foundation** 1300 858 584; adf.org.au **Alcoholics Anonymous** 1300 222 222; aa.org.au **The National Alcohol & Other Drug Hotline** 1800 250 015 **Counselling Online** counselling online.org.au **Quitline** (smoking) 137 848; quit.org.au **The National Gambling Helpline** 1800 858 858 **Gambling Help Online** gamblinghelponline.org.au

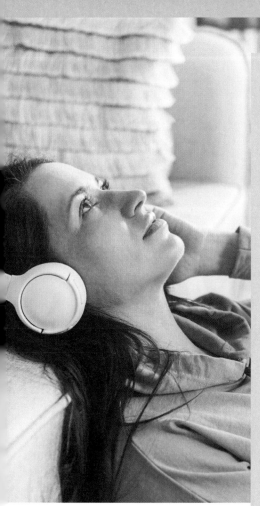

Wellbeing podcasts worth a listen

Tuning into a podcast is the perfect way to carve out some time for yourself, and perhaps learn a little more about your mental health and wellbeing. You can listen to podcasts while walking, on your daily commute, while cooking dinner or before you fall asleep. Have a listen to these Australian-produced wellness offerings for a healthy dose of information, inspiration and motivation.

WELLNESS WOMEN RADIO
Women's health experts Dr Ashleigh Bond and Dr Andrea Huddleston cover a range of female-specific topics, from thyroid health to childbirth and menopause.

NOT ALONE
Produced by Beyond Blue, this podcast profiles everyday Australians who share their journeys with anxiety, bullying, stress, isolation and healing to make an important point: you're not alone.

DEAR HEADSPACE
Meditation teachers answer questions on topics, such as work stress, relationships, body image and learning to say no.

BEING WELL
Produced by the Black Dog Institute, this podcast invites experts, advocates and inspiring Australians to share their insights around mental health.

GOOD MOURNING
Two women who unexpectedly lost their mums during lockdown speak to leading experts on grief, loss, trauma and mental health.

MINDFULLY
In partnership with mindfulness app Smiling Mind, this podcast explores how to apply the principles of mindfulness to the different areas of our lives.

LADIES, WE NEED TO TALK
Host Yumi Stynes tackles often taboo topics important to women, such as alcohol consumption, sexuality, birth trauma and burnout.

GREAT MINDS
Available in six languages, this podcast explores traditional meditation styles from around the world.

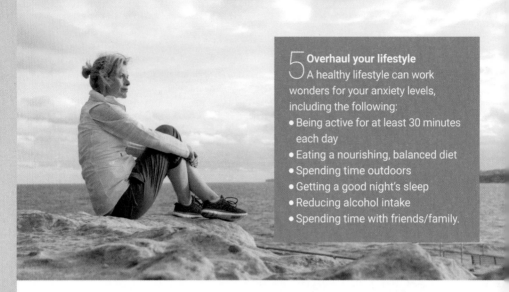

5 **Overhaul your lifestyle**
A healthy lifestyle can work wonders for your anxiety levels, including the following:
- Being active for at least 30 minutes each day
- Eating a nourishing, balanced diet
- Spending time outdoors
- Getting a good night's sleep
- Reducing alcohol intake
- Spending time with friends/family.

5 strategies for managing anxiety

Anxiety is the most common mental health disorder in Australia, affecting one in six people at some stage in their life. More than just stress or worry, anxious feelings don't easily go away and may not always have a clear cause. But there are ways to manage the symptoms. Every person's experience with anxiety is different, so try a few to see what works for you.

1 **Get to know your anxiety** If you can pinpoint the potential triggers behind your anxiety, you might identify the best ways to manage it. Keep a diary of each time you feel anxious and anything that may have contributed to it. Also learn to recognise the signs that your anxiety is increasing, such as feeling lethargic, getting worked up over small things, withdrawing socially or snapping at your partner.

2 **Challenge your worries** Avoiding situations that make you feel anxious can actually increase your anxiety over time. Instead, try challenging those worries in small ways. For example, if social events are your kryptonite, practise going out in smaller groups. If money matters make you anxious, sign up for an investing course.

3 **Practise slow breathing** When you're anxious, your breathing becomes fast and shallow, adding to the sense of panic and overwhelm. Try this simple exercise: place one hand on your chest and the other on your abdomen. Count to three as you breathe in slowly through your nose – you should feel your abdomen move but not your chest. Count to three as you breathe out slowly through your mouth. Repeat.

4 **Seek support** Confide in someone you trust, whether that's a friend or family member, your GP or a counsellor. Talk about how you're feeling and discuss potential anxiety triggers so your support crew can help you avoid or manage them. Ask them to look out for changes in your behaviour that you may not notice yourself.

For more information, visit Lifeline Australia; lifeline.org.au

How to do a mental health audit

We all have days when we feel flat, sad or just not like our usual selves. There can be a number of contributing factors that might cause these feelings, such as poor sleep, stress, hunger, interactions with other people, hormonal factors, medications, the weather, physical pain or a lack of exercise. Doing a daily check-in with yourself can help pinpoint any problematic feelings and their triggers, as well as highlight when you might need to seek help from a GP or healthcare professional. Use this checklist to make prioritising your mental health a regular part of your daily routine.

DATE

My stress level today (1 being not at all and 10 being extremely)

1   2   3   4   5   6   7   8   9   10

Today I feel...   (circle all that apply)

Calm   Motivated   Loved   Happy   Focused   Grateful   Energetic

Silly   Content   Tired   Lazy   Bored   Average   Depressed   Unmotivated

Lonely   Sad   Angry   Annoyed   Grumpy   Normal   Numb   Anxious

I started feeling this when...
_____
_____
_____

Current thoughts/concerns
_____
_____
_____

Today I...

☐ Drank 2L of water

☐ Moved my body

☐ Spent time outside

☐ Did something for me

☐ Connected with others

☐ Chose a relaxing activity

☐ Asked for help

☐ Went to bed on time

5 things I'm grateful for

1 _____

2 _____

3 _____

4 _____

5 _____

Tomorrow I'm looking forward to...
_____
_____

AUGUST
S	M	T	W	T	F	S
				1	2	3
4	5	6	7	8	9	10
11	12	13	14	15	16	17
18	19	20	21	22	23	24
25	26	27	28	29	30	31

SEPTEMBER
S	M	T	W	T	F	S
1	2	3	4	5	6	7
8	9	10	11	12	13	14
15	16	17	18	19	20	21
22	23	24	25	26	27	28
29	30					

OCTOBER
S	M	T	W	T	F	S
		1	2	3	4	5
6	7	8	9	10	11	12
13	14	15	16	17	18	19
20	21	22	23	24	25	26
27	28	29	30	31		

2 MONDAY

3 TUESDAY

4 WEDNESDAY INDIGENOUS LITERACY DAY

5 THURSDAY

6 FRIDAY

7 SATURDAY

> **EXPOSE YOUR BODY TO SUNLIGHT** each day to release endorphins, aka the happiness hormones. Sit outside, go for a walk or do some gardening – don't forget the SPF30!

8 SUNDAY

AUGUST
S	M	T	W	T	F	S
				1	2	3
4	5	6	7	8	9	10
11	12	13	14	15	16	17
18	19	20	21	22	23	24
25	26	27	28	29	30	31

SEPTEMBER
S	M	T	W	T	F	S
1	2	3	4	5	6	7
8	9	10	11	12	13	14
15	16	17	18	19	20	21
22	23	24	25	26	27	28
29	30					

OCTOBER
S	M	T	W	T	F	S
		1	2	3	4	5
6	7	8	9	10	11	12
13	14	15	16	17	18	19
20	21	22	23	24	25	26
27	28	29	30	31		

9 MONDAY

10 TUESDAY

11 WEDNESDAY

12 THURSDAY R U OK? DAY

13 FRIDAY

14 SATURDAY

> **IN TIMES OF STRESS,** do something creative. Try drawing, baking, jigsaws, sewing or playing a musical instrument to distract you from difficult thoughts or feelings or to help you process them.

15 SUNDAY

		AUGUST							SEPTEMBER							OCTOBER				
S	M	T	W	T	F	S	S	M	T	W	T	F	S	S	M	T	W	T	F	S
				1	2	3	1	2	3	4	5	6	7			1	2	3	4	5
4	5	6	7	8	9	10	8	9	10	11	12	13	14	6	7	8	9	10	11	12
11	12	13	14	15	16	17	15	16	17	18	19	20	21	13	14	15	16	17	18	19
18	19	20	21	22	23	24	22	23	24	25	26	27	28	20	21	22	23	24	25	26
25	26	27	28	29	30	31	29	30						27	28	29	30	31		

16 MONDAY EID MILAD UN NABI (PROPHET'S BIRTHDAY)

17 TUESDAY

18 WEDNESDAY

19 THURSDAY

September
2024

20 FRIDAY

21 SATURDAY

EAT MAGNESIUM-RICH FOODS to combat anxiety, depression and insomnia. Leafy green vegetables, legumes, nuts, seeds and wholegrains are good sources, as is tap water.

22 SUNDAY

	A U G U S T					
S	M	T	W	T	F	S
					1	2	3
4	5	6	7	8	9	10
11	12	13	14	15	16	17
18	19	20	21	22	23	24
25	26	27	28	29	30	31

	S E P T E M B E R					
S	M	T	W	T	F	S
1	2	3	4	5	6	7
8	9	10	11	12	13	14
15	16	17	18	19	20	21
22	23	24	25	26	27	28
29	30					

	O C T O B E R					
S	M	T	W	T	F	S
		1	2	3	4	5
6	7	8	9	10	11	12
13	14	15	16	17	18	19
20	21	22	23	24	25	26
27	28	29	30	31		

23 MONDAY KING'S BIRTHDAY (WA)

24 TUESDAY

25 WEDNESDAY

26 THURSDAY

September
2024

27 FRIDAY

28 SATURDAY

TUNE INTO THE BREAST CANCER TRIALS PODCAST to hear the latest research findings, treatment options as well as personal experiences. Available from your favourite podcast platform.

29 SUNDAY

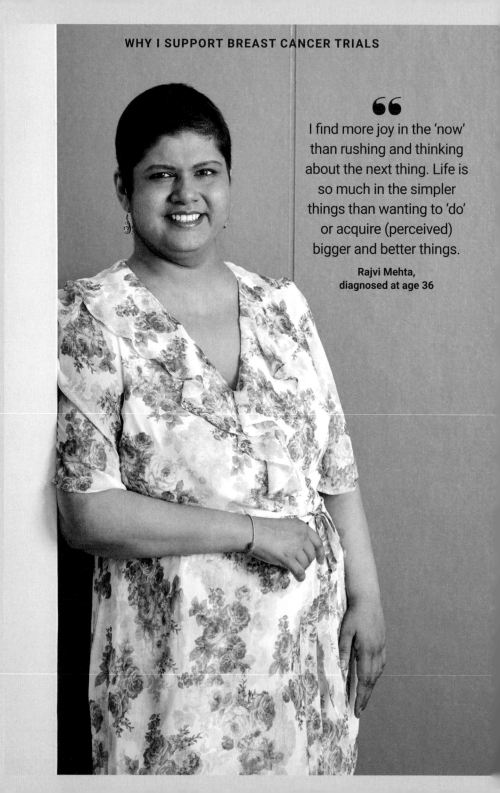

"

I find more joy in the 'now' than rushing and thinking about the next thing. Life is so much in the simpler things than wanting to 'do' or acquire (perceived) bigger and better things.

**Rajvi Mehta,
diagnosed at age 36**

let's talk about
BREAST HEALTH

In Australia, one in seven women will be diagnosed with breast cancer by the age of 85. With greater awareness and continued research, we can help create a more hopeful future for those affected.

There are a number of factors that can increase our chance of developing breast cancer. Some of these can be changed or modified, but others can't. Having one or more risk factors doesn't mean you will develop breast cancer, however, it's important to be aware of the contributing causes and make any lifestyle adjustments where possible.

PERSONAL FACTORS
There are a number of non-modifiable personal and physical factors that can influence a woman's risk for breast cancer. They include: getting older; being tall (our risk increases by 17 per cent for each additional 10cm above 175cm); and having a higher than average breast tissue density. The latter can be identified by mammogram.

GENETIC FACTORS
Having one or more blood relatives on your mother's or father's side who were diagnosed with breast cancer before the age of 50 increases your breast cancer risk. The inheritance of certain genetic mutations, such as BRCA1, BRCA2, PALB2 and CHEK2, can also increase the risk significantly.

REPRODUCTIVE FACTORS
If your first period started before the age of 12 or you experienced menopause after the age of 55, the risk of breast cancer increases. Having children later in life (after the age of 30) or not at all carries a similar risk. Again, these are factors often out of your control.

MEDICAL FACTORS
It's estimated that long-term use of menopausal hormone therapy (MHT) can increase our risk of breast cancer slightly, while there is a very slight risk when taking the oral contraceptive pill. There are also benefits for both, so it's important to discuss these with your doctor. A previous history of treatment for Hodgkin lymphoma and thyroid cancer may also increase your risk.

LIFESTYLE FACTORS
Some of our daily habits can make us more susceptible to breast cancer. For example, being overweight or obese and drinking alcohol have been shown to increase our risk, while smoking and eating processed meats may also contribute. The good news is we can make positive changes to reduce these factors and their associated risk.

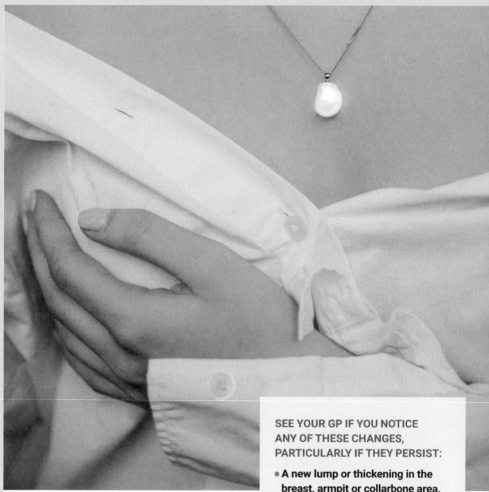

Signs & symptoms

The most obvious sign is finding a lump in the breast area. However, there are a number of other physical symptoms that may indicate breast cancer. Get to know the normal look and feel of your breasts and seek further advice if you notice any changes. In addition, book in for a screening mammogram every two years, which is free from the age of 40. The following changes may not always indicate breast cancer, however, you should always consult your doctor just to be sure.

SEE YOUR GP IF YOU NOTICE ANY OF THESE CHANGES, PARTICULARLY IF THEY PERSIST:

- **A new lump or thickening in the breast, armpit or collarbone area, especially if it's only on one side**
- **A change in breast size or shape**
- **Nipple changes, such as pain or tenderness, sores, crusting, ulceration, bleeding, redness or inversion**
- **Clear or bloody nipple discharge**
- **A change in the breast skin, such as puckering, scaliness, dimpling, redness or other colour variations**
- **An unusual tenderness, pain or swelling in the breast or armpit that doesn't go away.**

Helping a friend or loved one with breast cancer

Being diagnosed with breast cancer can take a huge emotional and physical toll on a person, as well as their friends and family. It can be difficult to know how best to support a loved one through their breast cancer journey, and they themselves may not always know what to ask for. But any help, support or kindness you offer will be invaluable as they navigate their way through the stages of diagnosis, treatment and recovery. Consider the following suggestions and strategies.

SUPPORTING A LOVED ONE

The number one thing you can do for your friend or family member is listen to their concerns, recognise their emotions and respond accordingly so they feel supported and hopeful about the future. Stay in touch regularly, but check that the timing suits them, as they may sometimes feel too tired to talk. Not every conversation needs to be about breast cancer – chatting about other things can be a welcome distraction! Avoid sharing the latest cure or treatment you've read about or burdening them with stories of other people with cancer – their journey is unique and they will be guided by their treatment team.

Some people find it difficult to ask for help, so try to identify tasks that you can assist with, whether that's cooking meals, hanging out the washing, driving them to appointments or looking after the children or pets. And acknowledge the significance of their diagnosis by staying on top of your own health checks and mammograms.

SUPPORTING A COLLEAGUE

Breast cancer treatment and diagnosis affects everyone differently – some women will want to continue working to maintain a sense of normalcy while others will need to take some time away. Ask if they want others to know about their diagnosis and how they would like this shared.

If you're their manager, establish their sick leave entitlements and discuss any other financial options or flexible working arrangements, if available. Don't be afraid to ask how they are feeling and if they need additional support in their role, and understand that both physical and mental impacts of breast cancer treatment can be long-lasting and that ongoing adjustments to work may be needed. Continue inviting them to meetings and events and explain there is no expectation for them to attend.

SUPPORT FOR YOU

It's very normal for partners, family members and friends of breast cancer patients to experience a range of emotions, from shock and sadness to anger and anxiety. While caring for your loved one, don't neglect your own health and wellbeing. Make time for exercise and self-care, and try to eat nutritious meals. Maintain family life as much as possible and inform your workplace or school of what is happening so they can support you as needed. Be kind to yourself and accept that you won't have all the answers. Ask for help when you need it by seeking counselling or help from organisations like Carers Australia or the government-supported Carer Gateway.

Metastatic breast cancer

Metastatic breast cancer, also known as advanced, secondary or stage four breast cancer, is the term given to a breast cancer that has spread to other parts of the body, such as the bones, liver, brain or lungs. It is diagnosed in about 4.6 per cent of women at the time of their first diagnosis, and in up to 15 per cent of women who were initially diagnosed with early stage breast cancer.

There is currently no cure for metastatic breast cancer, however, new and improved treatment options may be used to slow its progress, relieve symptoms and maintain quality of life. These treatments can include chemotherapy, hormonal therapy, targeted therapy, radiotherapy and surgery, and will depend on the type, location and size of the cancer and the potential side effects on the patient. These treatments can be highly effective in controlling the cancer, even if they cannot get rid of it entirely.

The emotional toll that women with metastatic breast cancer face, along with their loved ones, can be extensive. Consider seeking support and counselling to work through these challenges.

Hereditary breast cancer

Most people who develop breast cancer have had no previous family history of the disease. However, there is an increased risk if you do have a family history. The likelihood depends on the number of family members and the type of cancer they've had (not just breast cancer). As well as the risk that comes with having a close relative who has had breast cancer, approximately 5-10 per cent of breast cancers are caused by an inherited gene mutation, most commonly of the BRCA1 or BRCA2 genes. It's estimated that one in 400 Australian people have these genetic abnormalities, with a higher occurrence in people of Ashkenazi (European) Jewish heritage. Carrying a BRCA1 gene mutation comes with an approximate 70 per cent risk of developing breast cancer and a 44 per cent risk of developing ovarian cancer, while a BRCA2 mutation carries a 60 per cent and 15 per cent chance of breast or ovarian cancer respectively.

Have conversations with your family to determine any hereditary risk, after which you may consider genetic testing through a family cancer clinic. Typically, the person with the highest chance of testing positive for the gene is tested first (often the person who has had cancer), and then other family members can be tested if that person has a positive test. If positive, you'll be given a health plan of recommended steps to manage this risk.

Currently the most effective risk-reduction method for women with the BRCA1 and BRCA2 gene mutations is a double mastectomy – the removal of both healthy breasts. Removal of ovaries reduces the ovarian cancer risk, and also reduces breast cancer risk in premenopausal women.

THE BRCA-P CLINICAL TRIAL currently being conducted by Breast Cancer Trials is investigating if there is a less-invasive option to prevent BRCA1-associated breast cancer. For more information, visit breastcancertrials.org.au.

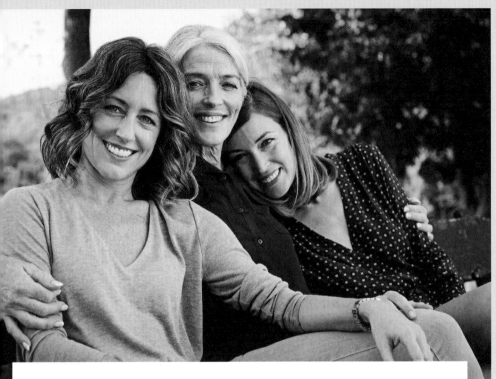

Why clinical trials matter

Breast cancer is now the most commonly diagnosed cancer in the world, with around 2.3 million people diagnosed globally each year. Its prevalence is certainly increasing here in Australia, but thankfully so too is the survival rate, and Breast Cancer Trials has played a significant role in this shift.

The treatments available to women and men diagnosed with breast cancer today are a direct result of the outcomes from clinical trials research. Clinical trials identify new treatment options, prevention strategies, diagnostic and detection tools and ways to lessen the physical, emotional and financial burden of breast cancer on patients.

There are different types of breast cancer and thus each person's diagnosis is unique to them. Factors such as the type, size and stage of the breast cancer, together with a woman's age and menopausal status, will influence her treatment plan. Our challenge, through clinical trials research, is to personalise treatment so that every person has the highest chance of long-term cure.

The researchers at Breast Cancer Trials have many important clinical trials currently underway to address this, including prevention of breast cancer in those who carry a genetic mutation, trials to identify new, targeted treatments for people with metastatic or early-stage breast cancer, and trials that seek to lessen the short and long-term side effects from treatment.

Sadly, nine women still lose their lives to breast cancer in Australia every day. Your support in buying this diary is critical in ensuring no more lives are cut short by this disease.

For more information, visit breastcancertrials.org.au

S	E	P	T	E	M	B	E	R
S	M	T	W	T	F	S
1	2	3	4	5	6	7
8	9	10	11	12	13	14
15	16	17	18	19	20	21
22	23	24	25	26	27	28
29	30					

O	C	T	O	B	E	R
S	M	T	W	T	F	S
		1	2	3	4	5
6	7	8	9	10	11	12
13	14	15	16	17	18	19
20	21	22	23	24	25	26
27	28	29	30	31		

N	O	V	E	M	B	E	R
S	M	T	W	T	F	S
					1	2
3	4	5	6	7	8	9
10	11	12	13	14	15	16
17	18	19	20	21	22	23
24	25	26	27	28	29	30

30 MONDAY

1 TUESDAY BREAST CANCER AWARENESS MONTH

2 WEDNESDAY

3 THURSDAY ROSH HASHANAH (JEWISH NEW YEAR)

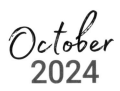

October
2024

4 FRIDAY

5 SATURDAY

6 SUNDAY DAYLIGHT SAVING TIME STARTS (ACT, NSW, SA, TAS, VIC)

SEPTEMBER

S	M	T	W	T	F	S
1	2	3	4	5	6	7
8	9	10	11	12	13	14
15	16	17	18	19	20	21
22	23	24	25	26	27	28
29	30					

OCTOBER

S	M	T	W	T	F	S
		1	2	3	4	5
6	7	8	9	10	11	12
13	14	15	16	17	18	19
20	21	22	23	24	25	26
27	28	29	30	31		

NOVEMBER

S	M	T	W	T	F	S
					1	2
3	4	5	6	7	8	9
10	11	12	13	14	15	16
17	18	19	20	21	22	23
24	25	26	27	28	29	30

7 MONDAY LABOUR DAY (ACT, NSW, SA), KING'S BIRTHDAY (QLD)

8 TUESDAY

9 WEDNESDAY

10 THURSDAY

11 FRIDAY

MANY BREAST CHANGES OCCUR in conjunction with hormonal fluctuations, such as while breastfeeding, menstruating or with menopause. See your GP if they persist.

12 SATURDAY YOM KIPPUR (JEWISH HOLY DAY)

13 SUNDAY

SEPTEMBER						
S	M	T	W	T	F	S
1	2	3	4	5	6	7
8	9	10	11	12	13	14
15	16	17	18	19	20	21
22	23	24	25	26	27	28
29	30					

OCTOBER						
S	M	T	W	T	F	S
		1	2	3	4	5
6	7	8	9	10	11	12
13	14	15	16	17	18	19
20	21	22	23	24	25	26
27	28	29	30	31		

NOVEMBER						
S	M	T	W	T	F	S
					1	2
3	4	5	6	7	8	9
10	11	12	13	14	15	16
17	18	19	20	21	22	23
24	25	26	27	28	29	30

14 MONDAY

15 TUESDAY

16 WEDNESDAY

17 THURSDAY

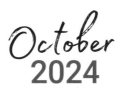

October
2024

18 FRIDAY

19 SATURDAY

IF YOU HAVE A FAMILY HISTORY of breast cancer, the iPrevent tool can help you better understand its relevance. Visit iPrevent.net.au.

20 SUNDAY

S	E	P	T	E	M	B	E	R
S	M	T	W	T	F	S
1	2	3	4	5	6	7
8	9	10	11	12	13	14
15	16	17	18	19	20	21
22	23	24	25	26	27	28
29	30					

O	C	T	O	B	E	R
S	M	T	W	T	F	S
		1	2	3	4	5
6	7	8	9	10	11	12
13	14	15	16	17	18	19
20	21	22	23	24	25	26
27	28	29	30	31		

N	O	V	E	M	B	E	R
S	M	T	W	T	F	S
					1	2
3	4	5	6	7	8	9
10	11	12	13	14	15	16
17	18	19	20	21	22	23
24	25	26	27	28	29	30

21 MONDAY

22 TUESDAY

23 WEDNESDAY

24 THURSDAY   ROYAL HOBART SHOW (TAS)

October
2024

25 FRIDAY

26 SATURDAY

> **REGULAR EXERCISE** lowers our breast cancer risk by approximately 20 per cent. Aim for 2.5 hours of moderate exercise or 1.5 hours of strenuous exercise each week.

27 SUNDAY

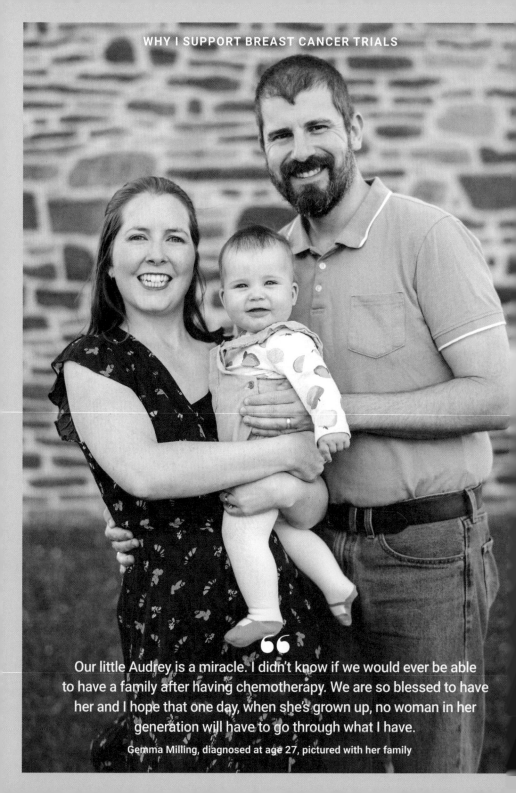

Our little Audrey is a miracle. I didn't know if we would ever be able to have a family after having chemotherapy. We are so blessed to have her and I hope that one day, when she's grown up, no woman in her generation will have to go through what I have.

Gemma Milling, diagnosed at age 27, pictured with her family

let's talk about
HEALTHY SKIN

No matter your age, taking care of your skin will help you feel good inside and out. From hydration and sun protection to tailor-made treatments, there are lots of ways to show your skin some love.

Affecting up to one in 10 adults and 30 per cent of children, eczema (also known as atopic dermatitis) is a chronic health condition that causes the skin to become dry, red, itchy and irritated. The symptoms can range from mild to moderate to debilitating.

LIVING WITH ECZEMA

Cause People with eczema have a skin barrier that is inefficient at keeping out environmental irritants and allergens, which results in an inflammatory response (redness, itchiness, dryness). The skin may also struggle to retain moisture, contributing to the dryness and irritation. Scratching the skin causes the release of more inflammatory chemicals, leading to a frustrating scratch-itch-scratch cycle. Eczema is often hereditary and many sufferers have other allergic conditions like asthma, hay fever or food allergy.

COMMON TRIGGERS
Eczema sufferers have various triggers that can make symptoms worse, including the following:

Household products or cosmetics containing perfumes, artificial colours, preservatives or soap

Sand, chlorine or grass

Carpet, wool or prickly fabrics

Viral or bacterial infections

Dust mites and animal fur or saliva

Heat or temperature changes

Stress

Appearance Eczema presents differently in children and adults. Babies will usually have flare-ups of redness, weeping and crusting around the face and neck area, while older children (aged 2-12) may experience dry skin around the neck, mouth, knees and elbows. Sometimes eczema comes on in adulthood, with symptoms similar to those of older children, albeit often more severe and widespread.

Treatment & management
While there is no cure for eczema, identifying the triggers and finding ways to manage them can help. Your GP or dermatologist can recommend measures to take based on your individual needs. Topical cortisone creams or ointments may be prescribed to help symptoms subside and reduce flare-ups, and in severe cases, oral medications or injections may be needed.

For more information, visit The Australasian College of Dermatologists; dermcoll.edu.au

10 healthy skin habits

You don't need to spend a fortune on cosmetic treatments or luxurious products to achieve glowing skin. Adopt these simple, low-maintenance techniques to maintain a healthy complexion and give your skin the care it deserves.

1 **MOISTURISE AFTER SHOWERING** Long baths or showers can strip the skin of essential oils, so moisturising will help replenish them. Moisturiser also boosts hydration, particularly important if your skin is dry or prone to inflammatory conditions like eczema or rosacea.

2 **REDUCE SKIN IRRITANTS** Perfumes, detergents and many other harmful chemicals can irritate or dry the skin, so where possible, look for gentle, fragrance-free, hypoallergenic soaps and cleansers, and wear gloves when washing up or working in the garden.

3 **LIMIT MAKE-UP** Wearing lots of make-up clogs the pores, resulting in blackheads and pimples. The use of too many skincare products can do the same thing. Keep it simple, don't forget your SPF and always remove your make-up before bed.

4 **EAT MORE FRUIT AND VEG** Aim for a variety, particularly those containing vitamin C (oranges, strawberries), vitamin E (avocados, spinach), betacarotene (carrots, sweet potato) and antioxidants (blueberries, leafy greens) to give your skin a healthy glow and repair signs of ageing.

6 **QUIT SMOKING** Smoking damages the skin's collagen and elastin layers and can contribute to the signs of ageing. Not to mention, it increases your risk of many cancers.

7 **STAY HYDRATED** Drinking the recommended eight cups (two litres) of water each day helps hydrate the skin and flushes out toxins to prevent acne. Find a vessel you enjoy drinking from, add herbs or lemon slices to your glass or alternate with herbal tea and sparkling water.

8 **CHECK USE-BY DATES** Using skincare products beyond their expiration date can compromise the skin barrier and lead to contamination, infection and acne. While not all skincare products come with expiry dates, as a general rule, cleansers, exfoliants, toners, moisturisers and serums should be replaced a year after opening. Preservative-free products tend to expire sooner.

9 **SLEEP WELL** If you're sleep deprived, your body produces excess amounts of the stress hormone cortisol, which can trigger itching, redness and inflammation. Aim to get eight hours of sleep each night to give the body a chance to repair and rejuvenate the skin cells.

5 **DRINK ALCOHOL IN MODERATION** Alcohol can be extremely dehydrating, and when consumed in excess, it can also cause bloating, puffiness, acne, redness and premature ageing in the skin. Limit your intake to see the benefits.

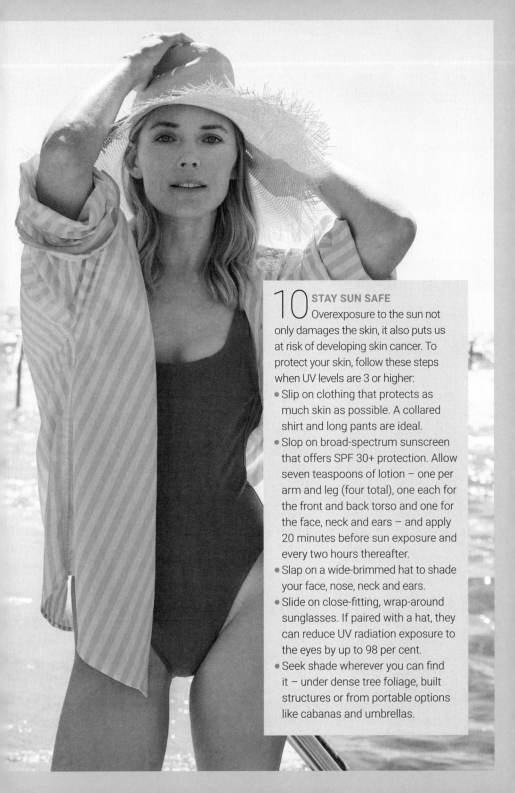

10 STAY SUN SAFE

Overexposure to the sun not only damages the skin, it also puts us at risk of developing skin cancer. To protect your skin, follow these steps when UV levels are 3 or higher:

- Slip on clothing that protects as much skin as possible. A collared shirt and long pants are ideal.
- Slop on broad-spectrum sunscreen that offers SPF 30+ protection. Allow seven teaspoons of lotion – one per arm and leg (four total), one each for the front and back torso and one for the face, neck and ears – and apply 20 minutes before sun exposure and every two hours thereafter.
- Slap on a wide-brimmed hat to shade your face, nose, neck and ears.
- Slide on close-fitting, wrap-around sunglasses. If paired with a hat, they can reduce UV radiation exposure to the eyes by up to 98 per cent.
- Seek shade wherever you can find it – under dense tree foliage, built structures or from portable options like cabanas and umbrellas.

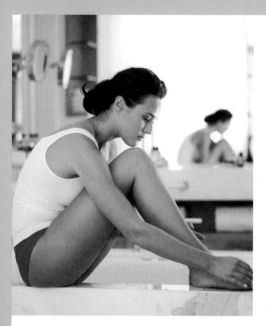

Monitor those spots

As well as practising sun safety whenever we spend time outdoors, we should make a habit of checking our skin for changes to existing freckles or moles as well as new spots. Use a full-length or handheld mirror when doing your checks, or ask a family member to help. And don't forget to examine all areas of your skin, not just those exposed to the sun, including your scalp, soles of the feet and between fingers and toes. Any changes in colour, size, texture or shape could be a sign of skin cancer and requires further examination by your GP. Here are the most common forms of skin cancer and what to look for.

TYPE	DESCRIPTION	LOOK OUT FOR
BASAL CELL CARCINOMA (BCC)	• The most common form of skin cancer, accounting for about 70 per cent of non-melanoma cases. • Usually grows slowly on parts of the body that have received high sun exposure.	• A pearly lump. • Dry, scaly area, which can either be shiny and pale or bright pink. • May ulcerate as it grows or look like a sore that isn't healing.
SQUAMOUS CELL CARCINOMA (SCC)	• Accounts for about 30 per cent of non-melanoma skin cancers in Australia. • Typically occurs on areas with high sun exposure. • Fast growing – over weeks/months.	• A thickened, red and scaly spot. • May be tender to the touch. • Can bleed easily, crust or ulcerate.
SUPERFICIAL SPREADING (TYPICAL) MELANOMA	• Melanoma can grow quickly and should be attended to as soon as possible. • Can appear on skin not normally exposed to the sun, and if left untreated, it can spread to other parts of the body.	• A flat spot or mole with an uneven border. • Can be blotchy and more than one colour. • Changes in size and shape; the spot may itch and bleed at times.
NODULAR MELANOMA	• An aggressive form that grows quickly and can become life-threatening in as little as six weeks.	• Raised to the touch. Firm, even colouring – they can be red, pink, brown or black.

For more information, visit Cancer Council Australia; cancer.org.au

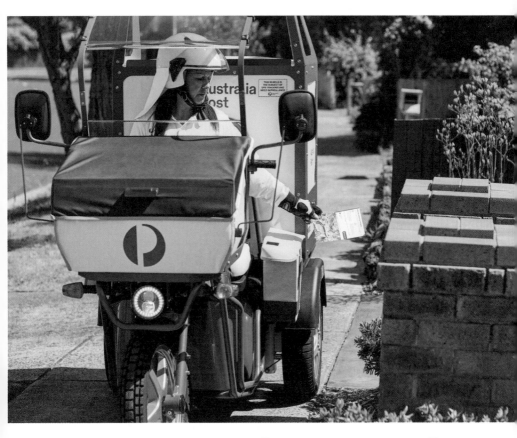

Delivering the Goods

By sending books to First Nations children, supporting mental wellbeing and raising funds in times of disaster, we're supporting communities in every corner of the country.

auspost.com.au

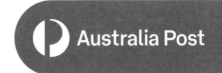

		OCTOBER				
S	M	T	W	T	F	S
		1	2	3	4	5
6	7	8	9	10	11	12
13	14	15	16	17	18	19
20	21	22	23	24	25	26
27	28	29	30	31		

		NOVEMBER				
S	M	T	W	T	F	S
					1	2
3	4	5	6	7	8	9
10	11	12	13	14	15	16
17	18	19	20	21	22	23
24	25	26	27	28	29	30

		DECEMBER				
S	M	T	W	T	F	S
1	2	3	4	5	6	7
8	9	10	11	12	13	14
15	16	17	18	19	20	21
22	23	24	25	26	27	28
29	30	31				

28 MONDAY AUSTRALIA'S BREAST CANCER DAY

29 TUESDAY

30 WEDNESDAY

31 THURSDAY HALLOWEEN

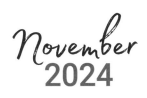

November
2024

1 FRIDAY DIWALI (HINDU, BUDDHIST, JAIN AND SIKH FESTIVAL)

2 SATURDAY

HELP CREATE A FUTURE where breast cancer no longer impacts lives by leaving a gift in your will to Breast Cancer Trials. Visit breastcancertrials. org.au for more information.

3 SUNDAY

		OCTOBER				
S	M	T	W	T	F	S
		1	2	3	4	5
6	7	8	9	10	11	12
13	14	15	16	17	18	19
20	21	22	23	24	25	26
27	28	29	30	31		

		NOVEMBER				
S	M	T	W	T	F	S
					1	2
3	4	5	6	7	8	9
10	11	12	13	14	15	16
17	18	19	20	21	22	23
24	25	26	27	28	29	30

		DECEMBER				
S	M	T	W	T	F	S
1	2	3	4	5	6	7
8	9	10	11	12	13	14
15	16	17	18	19	20	21
22	23	24	25	26	27	28
29	30	31				

4 MONDAY RECREATION DAY (TAS)

5 TUESDAY MELBOURNE CUP DAY (VIC)

6 WEDNESDAY

7 THURSDAY

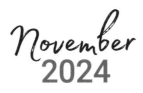

November
2024

8 FRIDAY

9 SATURDAY

10 SUNDAY

OCTOBER						
S	M	T	W	T	F	S
		1	2	3	4	5
6	7	8	9	10	11	12
13	14	15	16	17	18	19
20	21	22	23	24	25	26
27	28	29	30	31		

NOVEMBER						
S	M	T	W	T	F	S
					1	2
3	4	5	6	7	8	9
10	11	12	13	14	15	16
17	18	19	20	21	22	23
24	25	26	27	28	29	30

DECEMBER						
S	M	T	W	T	F	S
1	2	3	4	5	6	7
8	9	10	11	12	13	14
15	16	17	18	19	20	21
22	23	24	25	26	27	28
29	30	31				

11 MONDAY REMEMBRANCE DAY

12 TUESDAY

13 WEDNESDAY

14 THURSDAY

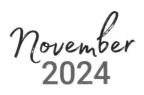

November
2024

15 FRIDAY

16 SATURDAY

> **REGULARLY EATING FAST FOODS** with a high glycaemic index (GI) has been linked to an increased risk of acne. Cut down on burgers, hot dogs, fries and soft drinks.

17 SUNDAY

OCTOBER						
S	M	T	W	T	F	S
		1	2	3	4	5
6	7	8	9	10	11	12
13	14	15	16	17	18	19
20	21	22	23	24	25	26
27	28	29	30	31		

NOVEMBER						
S	M	T	W	T	F	S
					1	2
3	4	5	6	7	8	9
10	11	12	13	14	15	16
17	18	19	20	21	22	23
24	25	26	27	28	29	30

DECEMBER						
S	M	T	W	T	F	S
1	2	3	4	5	6	7
8	9	10	11	12	13	14
15	16	17	18	19	20	21
22	23	24	25	26	27	28
29	30	31				

18 MONDAY

19 TUESDAY

20 WEDNESDAY

21 THURSDAY

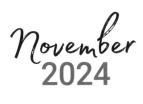

22 FRIDAY

23 SATURDAY

EASE SUNBURN
by running a bath.
Skip the bubble
bath, which can
irritate sunburnt
skin, and add
ground oats,
baking soda or
a cup of apple
cider vinegar to
lukewarm (not hot)
water. Pat skin dry.

24 SUNDAY

OCTOBER						
S	M	T	W	T	F	S
		1	2	3	4	5
6	7	8	9	10	11	12
13	14	15	16	17	18	19
20	21	22	23	24	25	26
27	28	29	30	31		

NOVEMBER						
S	M	T	W	T	F	S
					1	2
3	4	5	6	7	8	9
10	11	12	13	14	15	16
17	18	19	20	21	22	23
24	25	26	27	28	29	30

DECEMBER						
S	M	T	W	T	F	S
1	2	3	4	5	6	7
8	9	10	11	12	13	14
15	16	17	18	19	20	21
22	23	24	25	26	27	28
29	30	31				

25 MONDAY

26 TUESDAY

27 WEDNESDAY

28 THURSDAY

29 FRIDAY

30 SATURDAY

NEED A REASON TO GO SCREEN-FREE? Blue light from computers and phones may be harmful to the skin, contributing to loss of firmness and an increase in visible lines.

1 SUNDAY

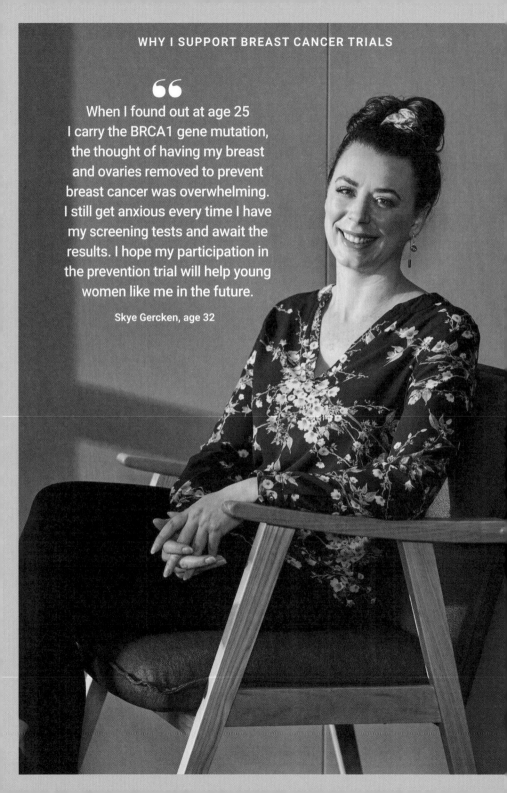

" When I found out at age 25
I carry the BRCA1 gene mutation,
the thought of having my breast
and ovaries removed to prevent
breast cancer was overwhelming.
I still get anxious every time I have
my screening tests and await the
results. I hope my participation in
the prevention trial will help young
women like me in the future.

Skye Gercken, age 32

let's talk about LIFESTYLE

Life can be busy and overwhelming at times. Put steps in place at home, at work and in your daily routine to prioritise relaxation, healthy balance and most of all, find enjoyment in every day.

When we're stressed and juggling multiple tasks at once, finding time to relax can seem like an unachievable dream, but this is actually when we need it most. Practising relaxation techniques for just five minutes a day can help reduce anxiety, promote better sleep and increase immunity. Different relaxation techniques appeal to different people, so try a few options and rate each out of 10 to find your best fit.

MEDITATION Take a few minutes to sit quietly and focus on your breathing, allowing thoughts to come and go and tuning out the sounds around you. Try a guided app like Smiling Mind or Headspace to get the hang of it. **Score:** _____

POSITIVE AFFIRMATIONS Repeat positive statements in your mind to counter negative thoughts or worries. For example, "I can do this", "This too shall pass" or "I am safe and in control". **Score:** _____

LAUGHTER Watch a funny movie, go to a comedy show or laugh with friends to prompt your body's release of natural feel-good chemicals. **Score:** _____

EXERCISE Just 10 minutes of exercise will release endorphins to help put your mind at ease. Try rhythmic activities like rowing, running or swimming. **Score:** _____

VISUALISATION Using your senses, imagine a peaceful scene: a beach, forest, pool or trickling river. How does it smell, look, sound and feel? **Score:** _____

YOGA The flowing movements and rhythmic breathing of yoga can help calm the mind and relieve muscle tension. Take a class or online tutorial. **Score:** _____

DEEP BREATHING Close your eyes, drop your shoulders and breathe in slowly through your nose for a count of five, then breathe out for a count of five. Repeat until the stress begins to ebb away. **Score:** _____

MUSIC THERAPY Listen to or play music to reset your mind. Try upbeat tunes to increase motivation and optimism, and soft, slow tunes to de-stress. **Score:** _____

SELF-CARE Do something that makes you feel good, whether it's gardening, lighting a candle, meeting a friend for coffee or reading a magazine. **Score:** _____

6 ways to enjoy a healthy festive season

There's nothing like the end of the year to suddenly fill your calendar with work functions, family gatherings and social catch-ups. While it can be easy to overindulge during the silly season, there are ways to enjoy yourself without losing track of your healthy habits. Read on for our six-step festive season survival plan.

1 OPT FOR LIGHT STARTERS
Deep-fried canapes and pastries can increase your intake of salt, trans fats and saturated fats. Choose lighter options like grilled calamari, mini vegetable frittatas or a grazing board of dips, cheese, wholegrain crackers, marinated vegetables and olives.

2 ADD SOME COLOUR TO YOUR PLATE
Salads are perfect for summer parties, where guests are often asked to bring a dish. Vegetable sides are also an easy, inexpensive way to round out a meal. Fill at least half your plate with vegetables, from chargrilled corn, to roasted pumpkin, steamed greens or leafy salads.

3 GRILL YOUR PROTEIN
Cooking on the barbecue requires minimal oil and less time to cook, meaning the nutrients and flavours stay intact. Swap sausages, which tend to be high in salt, for lean lamb, pork cutlets, steak, chicken or mushrooms for a meat-free alternative.

4 HAVE YOUR CAKE
Apply the everything-in-moderation rule to dessert and treat yourself for a special occasion. If you'd prefer something on the healthier end of the sweet scale, try fruit-

5 CELEBRATE SEAFOOD
Guaranteed to wow a crowd, fish and seafood contain protein, zinc and omega-3 fatty acids. Serve prawns and oysters with a zingy vinaigrette, barbecue fish whole with fresh herbs and a squeeze of lemon or cook mussels in a delicious garlic or tomato-based broth.

based or low-sugar desserts. Think grilled stone fruit, oat-based crumbles, poached pears, fruit sorbet or coconut chia pudding.

6 EMBRACE MOCKTAILS
Watch your alcohol intake by opting for refreshing mocktails alternated with water. Use unsweetened fruit juice, soda water or

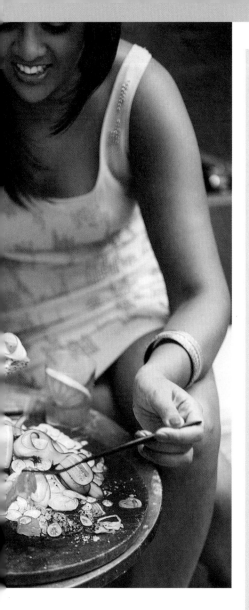

Enjoy the slow life

As the year comes to an end, your stress levels may be at an all-time high. But there is a way to opt out of this busyness and enjoy a more relaxed and purposeful approach to life – it's called slow living. This lifestyle philosophy is all about finding joy in life's simple pleasures. Try introducing some of these strategies and slow-living habits to live a less hurried life.

Take one slow day a week, where you don't schedule any appointments, activities or big errands. Instead, enjoy hobbies or pursuits you don't normally have time for – it might be having a picnic, reading a book in bed, playing a board game or baking a cake.

Stress less about mess by decluttering your home of non-essentials and introducing some streamlined storage solutions. No more rummaging through drawers, cupboards or shelves in search of misplaced items.

Rush less and re-train your brain to enjoy the journey as much as the destination. Leave the car at home and walk, cycle or catch public transport so you can take in the sights and sounds around you.

Prioritise family connection by enjoying meals together, greeting each other with hugs and kisses, having one-on-one conversations and sharing hobbies.

Plan holidays that revolve around rest and relaxation. Head outdoors to explore at your leisure rather than filling days with a long list of activities set to a regimented schedule.

sparkling water as a base, and add fresh herbs, berries, stone fruit, lime wedges or lemon slices, plus lots of ice.

And remember, there are no 'bad' foods. Enjoy this time with friends and family, and if you do overindulge, you can easily return to your healthy habits tomorrow.

Working from home tips

The Covid pandemic saw many Australians transition to working from home (WFH), and approximately 46 per cent have continued to do so since. For some, the advantages of working remotely (no commute, less office distractions, greater flexibility) outweigh the disadvantages. However, it's important we don't sacrifice our health in the quest for greater autonomy. Consider these ideas to care for your mind and body while WFH.

GET READY FOR WORK AS USUAL
Continue the routine of waking, showering, eating breakfast and getting dressed for work (albeit in casual attire) so you can start the day in the right headspace.

SET CLEAR BOUNDARIES
Working from home doesn't mean you should be on call 24/7. Have a regular start and finish time, with scheduled breaks, and communicate this with colleagues and family members, so they have a clear idea of when you will be available to them.

HAVE A DEDICATED WORKSPACE
Set up an area in your home that's reserved for work only, preferably not your bedroom or a living space shared by others. Make sure

STAY CONNECTED WITH YOUR CO-WORKERS
Social interactions reduce stress levels, boost productivity and help us feel less isolated. Schedule virtual check-ins with workmates each day, pick up the phone to chat through your progress rather than emailing or plan a weekly lunch or coffee catch-up for important face-to-face time.

MOVE OFTEN
Exercise has huge benefits for our health and wellbeing, so plan time in your day to do some, whether that's before work, during your lunch break or after work. Also try to get up from your desk at least once an hour – stand for phone calls, take a meeting while walking around the block or do some stretches while the kettle boils.

this work area is well lit and ergonomically set up to avoid neck, back or eye strain (see safeworkaustralia.gov.au for tips).

TAKE A PROPER LUNCH BREAK
Being close to the kitchen might see you grazing on unhealthy snacks all day, or alternatively, you may forget to eat entirely. Schedule in time to have lunch away from your desk; prepare it the night before to avoid reaching for less-healthy options.

BASK IN THE FLEXIBILITY
One of the perks of working remotely is greater productivity, so you can attend to personal errands or household tasks without the guilt. Fold washing while listening to a presentation, duck out to your child's school assembly in between meetings or make a start on dinner before moving on to your next work task.

SWITCH OFF AT THE END OF THE DAY
Once you've clocked off for the day, turn your phone to silent or switch off message notifications so you're not tempted to keep working. Make sure you've disconnected from all devices one hour before going to bed for a quality night's sleep.

THE AUSTRALIAN
Women's Weekly

A whole year of enjoyment

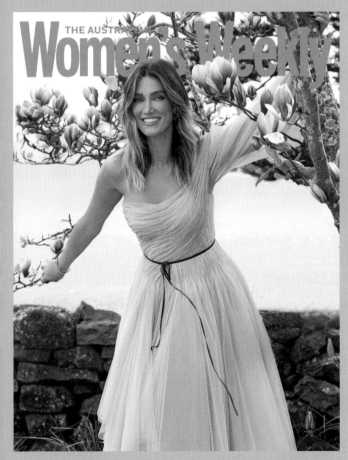

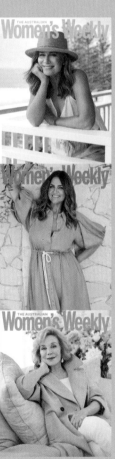

NOVEMBER						
S	M	T	W	T	F	S
					1	2
3	4	5	6	7	8	9
10	11	12	13	14	15	16
17	18	19	20	21	22	23
24	25	26	27	28	29	30

DECEMBER						
S	M	T	W	T	F	S
1	2	3	4	5	6	7
8	9	10	11	12	13	14
15	16	17	18	19	20	21
22	23	24	25	26	27	28
29	30	31				

JANUARY						
S	M	T	W	T	F	S
			1	2	3	4
5	6	7	8	9	10	11
12	13	14	15	16	17	18
19	20	21	22	23	24	25
26	27	28	29	30	31	

2 MONDAY

3 TUESDAY

4 WEDNESDAY

5 THURSDAY

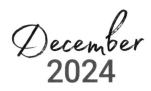

December
2024

6 FRIDAY

7 SATURDAY

8 SUNDAY

		NOVEMBER				
S	M	T	W	T	F	S
					1	2
3	4	5	6	7	8	9
10	11	12	13	14	15	16
17	18	19	20	21	22	23
24	25	26	27	28	29	30

		DECEMBER				
S	M	T	W	T	F	S
1	2	3	4	5	6	7
8	9	10	11	12	13	14
15	16	17	18	19	20	21
22	23	24	25	26	27	28
29	30	31				

		JANUARY				
S	M	T	W	T	F	S
			1	2	3	4
5	6	7	8	9	10	11
12	13	14	15	16	17	18
19	20	21	22	23	24	25
26	27	28	29	30	31	

9 MONDAY

10 TUESDAY

11 WEDNESDAY

12 THURSDAY

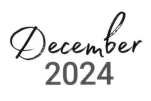

December
2024

13 FRIDAY

14 SATURDAY

> **FIND CREATIVE WAYS** to reduce the financial impact of Christmas. Send e-cards, trial Secret Santa for gift-giving or ask others to bring a plate towards a shared meal.

15 SUNDAY

NOVEMBER

S	M	T	W	T	F	S
					1	2
3	4	5	6	7	8	9
10	11	12	13	14	15	16
17	18	19	20	21	22	23
24	25	26	27	28	29	30

DECEMBER

S	M	T	W	T	F	S
1	2	3	4	5	6	7
8	9	10	11	12	13	14
15	16	17	18	19	20	21
22	23	24	25	26	27	28
29	30	31				

JANUARY

S	M	T	W	T	F	S
			1	2	3	4
5	6	7	8	9	10	11
12	13	14	15	16	17	18
19	20	21	22	23	24	25
26	27	28	29	30	31	

16 MONDAY

17 TUESDAY

18 WEDNESDAY

19 THURSDAY

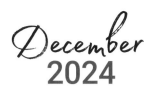

December
2024

20 FRIDAY

21 SATURDAY

FEELING TENSE?
Take a moment to correct your posture. Pull your shoulders back, straighten your spine and hold your head high with your chin up.

22 SUNDAY

NOVEMBER

S	M	T	W	T	F	S
					1	2
3	4	5	6	7	8	9
10	11	12	13	14	15	16
17	18	19	20	21	22	23
24	25	26	27	28	29	30

DECEMBER

S	M	T	W	T	F	S
1	2	3	4	5	6	7
8	9	10	11	12	13	14
15	16	17	18	19	20	21
22	23	24	25	26	27	28
29	30	31				

JANUARY

S	M	T	W	T	F	S
			1	2	3	4
5	6	7	8	9	10	11
12	13	14	15	16	17	18
19	20	21	22	23	24	25
26	27	28	29	30	31	

23 MONDAY

24 TUESDAY CHRISTMAS EVE

25 WEDNESDAY CHRISTMAS DAY

26 THURSDAY BOXING DAY, PROCLAMATION DAY (SA), FIRST DAY OF HANUKKAH

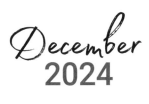

December
2024

27 FRIDAY

28 SATURDAY

> **AS THE YEAR COMES TO AN END,** write a list of your biggest health wins over the past 12 months, and what you'd like to work on in 2025.

29 SUNDAY

	NOVEMBER					
S	M	T	W	T	F	S
			1	2	3	4
5	6	7	8	9	10	11
12	13	14	15	16	17	18
19	20	21	22	23	24	25
26	27	28	29	30		

	DECEMBER					
S	M	T	W	T	F	S
31					1	2
3	4	5	6	7	8	9
10	11	12	13	14	15	16
17	18	19	20	21	22	23
24	25	26	27	28	29	30

	JANUARY					
S	M	T	W	T	F	S
	1	2	3	4	5	6
7	8	9	10	11	12	13
14	15	16	17	18	19	20
21	22	23	24	25	26	27
28	29	30	31			

30 MONDAY

31 TUESDAY NEW YEAR'S EVE

1 WEDNESDAY NEW YEAR'S DAY

2 THURSDAY

January
2025

3 FRIDAY

4 SATURDAY

ENJOY SUMMER IN A SAFE WAY. Plan beach swims when the UV index is 3 or below, wear a hat, sunscreen and sun-protective clothing outdoors and drink more water on hot days.

5 SUNDAY

Notes

Notes

Notes

THE AUSTRALIAN WOMEN'S

Health Diary ®

Editor: Tiffany Dunk

Art & Picture Director: Ellen Erickson

Writer & Copy Editor: Stephanie Hope

BCT Diary Manager: Julie Callaghan

BCT Diary Marketing: Belinda Carrall

Breast Cancer Trials (BCT)

1800 423 444; breastcancertrials.org.au

diaryenquiries@bctrials.org.au

The Australian Women's Health Diary®
is produced by the publishers of
The Australian Women's Weekly on
behalf of Breast Cancer Trials.

THE AUSTRALIAN Women's Weekly

Editor-in-Chief: Nicole Byers

Chief Executive Officer: Jane Huxley

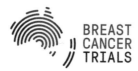

BREAST
CANCER
TRIALS